FULLY NOURISHED

The following words come from early readers—women who've battled diet rules, body shame, and the lie that their worth is tied to their weight. Their reflections, insights, and encouragements reflect the heart of Fully Nourished: *Real freedom isn't found in our performance but in our pursuit of Jesus. I pray their words remind you that you're not alone and that grace is already rewriting your story.*

"*Fully Nourished* is a refreshing, faith-based guide to breaking free from the dieting mindset. It beautifully weaves biblical truth with practical insights, helping you not only find freedom with food but also embrace your body with grace and gratitude. If you're ready to invite God into your health journey, let go of guilt, and see yourself through his eyes, this book is a must-read!"

Ginger Perkins

"Brandice gently guides us through eating challenges, giving us practical advice on how to deal with them, change our mindset, and draw closer to God in the process. Each chapter had steps I could take right away toward improving my eating habits, mindset, and overall health. I was excited to try each suggestion and see how they worked for me. The whole book has helped me learn to look at food in a more positive light. I'll return to it again and again as new challenges arise. Brandice has covered it all."

Rebecca Masney

"Most of us have been there: buying another diet book because all 943 we've accumulated have failed us. This will be the last one you'll ever need, not because it's another diet book but because it will address the root issues you've been avoiding or are scared to face. This book will teach you, step-by-step and chapter-by-chapter, that with God's help, you can embark on a journey full of hope, love, and healthy choices rather than going, yet again, on a diet roller coaster counting numbers, whether calories, macros, or pounds. May this book bless you and heal you from the inside out, whether you meet or find God for the first time or rekindle your relationship with him."

Elmaret Fourie

"Brandice has a true heart for God and for everyone she helps through their struggles with weight, self-esteem, and their walk with the Lord. *Fully Nourished* gives you the tools you need to look at food in a healthier way, to learn who you are in Christ, and to strengthen your relationship with God. It is not some strict diet to follow but a healthy approach to real-life struggles with tools to use for real lifestyle change—physically, emotionally, mentally, and spiritually."

Patti L.

"So grateful for the perspective Brandice has! This book just spoke to me in so many ways and really made me think about why I make certain choices and how to change them. Having the Christian perspective is so important to me, and *Fully Nourished* helped guide me toward appreciating what I can do through Christ!"

Jodi White

"'No one ever taught me how to navigate my fears and failures without food. And because eating was my best attempt at self-care, it became my number one coping mechanism.' That is one of my favorite quotes from *Fully Nourished* because that is me too! I used to think what I needed was to cut out all sugar from my diet or restrict some other aspect of my food intake. *Fully Nourished* is teaching me what the source of the problem is, not to just fix the symptoms. It's a journey that is moving me closer to Jesus. Practical steps into food freedom! Practical steps to lasting change!"

Nancy A.

"*Fully Nourished* is full of the practical wisdom of seeking God to fill your heart and making decisions that will lead to a healthy, sustainable lifestyle. Brandice shares her journey of learning her actual value and how to become grateful in the now while enjoying her progress toward her goals. This book explores learning how to reject the diet mindset while aligning your beliefs with God's Word. It is transformational and brings a sense of relief that frees you up to move forward confidently toward a healthy you. My life is being forever changed as I apply the fantastic information found within the pages of this book."

Jennifer Bradley

FULLY NOURISHED

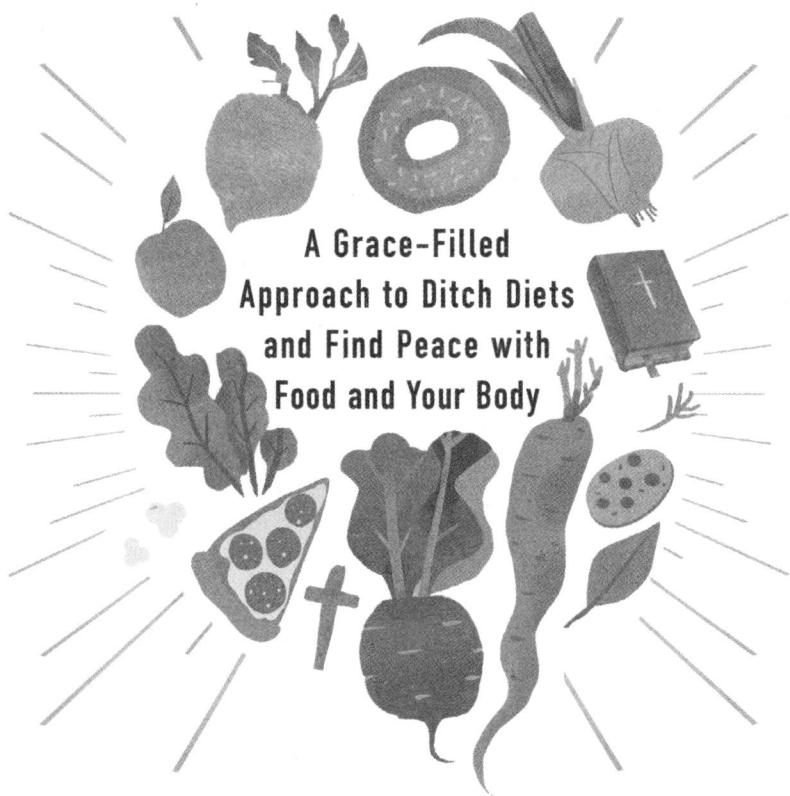

A Grace-Filled
Approach to Ditch Diets
and Find Peace with
Food and Your Body

BRANDICE LARDNER

Revell
a division of Baker Publishing Group
Grand Rapids, Michigan

Published by Revell
a division of Baker Publishing Group
Grand Rapids, Michigan
RevellBooks.com

Printed in the United States of America

Library of Congress Cataloging-in-Publication Data
Names: Lardner, Brandice, 1977– author
Title: Fully nourished : a grace-filled approach to ditch diets and find peace
   with food and your body / Brandice Lardner.
Description: Grand Rapids, Michigan : Revell, a division of Baker Publishing
   Group, [2026] | Includes bibliographical references.
Identifiers: LCCN 2025023260 | ISBN 9780800747039 (paperback) | ISBN
   9780800747930 (casebound) | ISBN 9781493452767 (ebook)
Subjects: LCSH: Food—Religious aspects—Christianity | Nutrition—
   Religious aspects—Christianity | Human body—Religious aspects—
   Christianity | Health—Religious aspects—Christianity
Classification: LCC BR115.N87 L373 2026 | DDC 241/.68—dc23/eng/20250801
LC record available at https://lccn.loc.gov/2025023260

Cover design by Lindy Kasler

The author is represented by the literary agency of The Blythe Daniel Agency Inc.

Baker Publishing Group publications use paper produced from sustainable forestry practices and postconsumer waste whenever possible.

26   27   28   29   30   31   32   7   6   5   4   3   2   1

To the woman weary from striving who knows Jesus is the answer but wonders how to begin—may this book be your gentle guide toward grace, freedom, and a deeper walk with him, showing you how to live his truth in practical, life-changing ways.

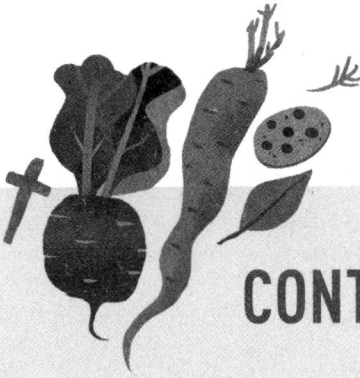

CONTENTS

INTRODUCTION

"Lord, let this time be different," I prayed.

I sat at the kitchen table, hovering over my latest diet book as if simply reading its black-and-white words would lead to my Cinderella story. I'll be honest; I skimmed past the science-y stuff and went right to my future—the list of "good" and "bad" foods. Nothing surprising . . . protein was in; tasty was out.

Just as I mourned the appearance of ice cream on the "don't eat" list, a chocolatey blob of my "last supper" of rocky road plopped onto the crisp, smooth, white page. I tried to wipe it clean, but then my vigorous scrubbing started to muddy the page, marking an ironic first sign of defeat.

It wasn't the first time something like this had happened. All my diet books were adorned with not only yellow highlighter but also coffee drips and ketchup smudges—glaring signs that I was never *really* ready to give up those favorite foods. Sigh. But I never saw the truth. I kept thinking, *If only I can find the right diet,* then *I'll finally hold the key to unlock the heavy door that's kept me trapped.*

If history repeated itself, this "new" book with the same old "eat this, don't eat that" approach would be gathering dust by month's end. "Why does it seem like everybody else is able to stick to a diet and lose weight but me?" I moaned. Thoughts of failure crushed my dreams, and I decided I might as well eat more ice cream, since I already knew how this was going to end.

But this diet disaster wasn't my fault. And if you can relate to those chocolate smudges, I promise it's not yours either. You don't *want* to trip up, but you've been *set up*.

Think about this: What happened the last time you tried and face-planted on a diet? You likely blamed yourself. It was *your* lack of self-control, *your* inability to follow the food plan, *your* gravitational pull to the drive-thru after soccer practice that led to your utter defeat. Not once did you consider that the diet did it.

Neither did I.

The Real Reason Diets Don't Work

The first time I went on a diet I was a rockstar.

I meticulously followed the food plan and ate dry tuna and cottage cheese as if it were the meal my mom made me on special occasions. I skipped the carbs and anything with notable calories. It went okay for quite some time. Months, even. Then something broke. I ate one. I don't even recall what that *one* was, but that deviation swept my feet out from under me. I tried to stop, but it felt like I had been trying to hold a beach ball underwater—every craving denied, meal avoided, and daydream about anything and everything chocolate resurfaced, and I engaged in an epic pantry raid.

Because I thought *I* was the weak link, I decided to try another diet. But this new plan declared dairy was the latest dietary villain. In fact, dairy was the reason I had acne, brain fog, and a random hair growing out of my chin. Now I had yet another food group to add to my "don't you dare eat that" list.

Diet by diet, food list by food list, the litany of things I shouldn't have continued to grow. It felt like there was nothing left I could eat. But that didn't mean I stopped thinking about all the foods I'd left behind—they were everywhere! Foods I hadn't noticed before seemed to pop up in the most unusual places when I was least expecting them.

My life was wholly wrapped up in what I ate, and the tug-of-war between "Should I eat . . . or not?" sucked the life out of me. I began to stay home to avoid social gatherings for fear of some "fattening" food attaching itself to my hips. The times I did brave the caloric unknown, I'd eat like a picture of perfect health only to go home and unleash myself on a box of cereal. I was exhausted and overwhelmed and felt like I'd never be able to get my diet right.

But I didn't have a character defect. What I had was a deficient skill set. No one had ever taught me how to navigate my fears and failures without food. And because eating was my best attempt at self-care, it became my number one coping mechanism.

Diets left me swallowed by my fears and failures. They've failed me—and you—because their arbitrary rules wobble and waver on the foundation of human thinking. What's in and out changes faster than we can follow, leaving us confused, defeated, and probably a bit more overweight. But the biggest reason diets don't work is because food was never the problem.

The Elephant in the Room

Did you flinch a bit just now, when I said that food was not the real problem? You may resist that thought because you feel like you've played a leading role in your food struggles, and that the primary source of your angst is how much you love to eat those so-called forbidden foods. The pantry calls your name when you're the only one awake, and you cherish those moments when you can finally treat yourself. It's you and the food, and that's all you can see. But there's so much more at play.

You have a story with food, and not all of it is broken.

When you were a baby, you cried for milk because you were hungry. When you were a toddler, you pushed away even the tastiest treat when your tummy was full and, sometimes, you even forgot about your Easter candy.

But you got older and life happened. You had a hard breakup, and the mac and cheese soothed your soul. You didn't get invited to the party, and you took out your frustration on a bag of chips.

You found solace in food, and it started to show. Bit by bit, your clothes got tighter and tighter, until you decided it was time to do something about it. That something was a diet. Food scales and calorie counts entered the scene and, restriction by restriction, your relationship with food got wrecked.

You tried to avoid eating things you "shouldn't," and the ice cream you once pushed away began to feel *pulled away*. It's all been exhausting, and you feel addicted to sweets and treats and crunchy snacks.

That's the nature of forbidden fruit—we want what we can't have, and, as you've probably noticed, the enemy capitalizes on it so he can lock our eyes on the problem rather than the Solution.

It's not about the food. It's about what you want food to do for you . . . that only God can. He can soothe every hurt and heal every wound when you let him in.

Are you ready to let the Lord guide and direct you to food freedom? This kind of freedom begins where self-sufficiency ends. It's not about perfect eating or cutting out entire food groups—it's about peace. Peace with food. Peace with your body. And peace with your heavenly Father.

Food freedom is about living nourished in body and spirit, no longer controlled by cravings, guilt, or shame. It's not the absence of struggle but the presence of grace.

The Journey We're About to Take Together

This book utilizes concepts I've used to coach thousands of women toward food freedom, all in a step-by-step guide. Each chapter builds on the previous concepts you've been taught while setting the stage for the next. Think of *Fully Nourished* as your personal guide—one that will encourage you to go at your own pace but also cheer you on to keep moving forward.

To get the most out of this book, I encourage you to read a chapter and then take some time (at least a week) to practice the concepts you've been taught before moving on.

Step 1: Read the chapter.

Step 2: Learn the action step (habit).

Step 3: Practice your new habit.

Step 4: Move on to the next chapter.

Now, before I spread out the map and ponder the journey with you, I'm reminded of my own propensity to flip to the back of the book. You know, the part where all the pieces seem to come together? I know how tempting it is to jump to the last step, but I am going to ask you to hang tight with me.

As mentioned, each chapter intentionally builds upon the one before it. If you were to skip ahead and dig in to your goals and

BETTER TOGETHER

Fully Nourished is all about simplifying your journey to food freedom. However, knowing when you need a support team is wisdom; don't hesitate to reach out to a Christian counselor or registered dietitian for guidance.

Also, as in any venture, we're better together! Now would be a great time to connect with a friend or Bible study group and ask them to join you. The camaraderie and support of a group will exponentially increase the likelihood of you completing your journey through this book (and theirs too).

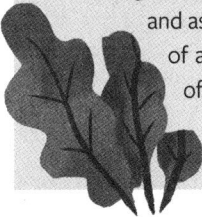

values without *first* fully understanding your worth and value outside of your performance and appearance, you'd only affirm your old thinking patterns. To find your peace in the process, take the time to follow the path. By its end, you'll be equipped to:

- Stop defining your value by how you eat and develop better self-worth.
- Feel grateful for your body—where you are *today*—without giving up on your weight loss goals.
- Have a mind that doesn't obsess over food and has room to enjoy the blessings God has given you.
- Enjoy what you eat mindfully, with a peace-filled heart.
- Stop thinking about food when you're not physically hungry.

Isn't it exciting to think that this struggle you've had, possibly for decades (like me), has felt impossible to overcome only because you've been using the wrong tools? What if the diet approach has been like swinging a hammer at your eating and body image—when what you really needed was the loving, steady shaping of the Lord? What if his still, small voice is what will gently mold and chisel you into a woman who walks in total freedom?

Are you ready? Let's start walking toward food freedom together.

— FULLY NOURISHED PRACTICE PAGES —

Visit https://GraceFilledPlate.com/fnbonus/ to download your free habit tracker. Print it out and keep it handy; you'll find it a helpful tool for each new habit.

Also included is a Scripture writing journal, which I'll prompt you to use each chapter to help keep your new habit and Jesus-first focus front and center.

You can also download printable Scripture cards for each chapter to display around your home, as well as a few other printable resources that will come in handy on your journey.

1

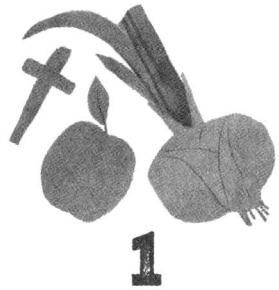

DON'T START FROM A DEFICIT

Give thanks in all circumstances; for this is the will of God in Christ Jesus for you.

1 Thessalonians 5:18

It was Saturday morning and time for my weekly weigh-in and measuring. I put on my workout clothes, pulled out my pink measuring tape, and headed to the scale. I was anxious to see my results because I'd worked *really* hard that week, and I had a feeling I'd finally made some notable progress. I took a deep breath and eased onto the scale, feeling like I was waiting for a judge and jury to return with a verdict.

And then it came. The verdict was not in my favor.

I stepped off the scale as a sense of panic rose from my stomach. Seeing that higher number felt like a punch to the gut. This isn't possible, I argued with myself. I've been doing so well—prepping my meals, going to the gym three days a week, and even eating vegetables for breakfast (breakfast!).

I reset the scale and stepped on it again. The exact same number stared back at me. My heart sank. I was so sure I'd lost at least a few pounds. *What a waste*, I fumed. *I give up.* Food and weight had always been my nemesis. Why had I expected anything different?

Can you relate? Have you been in this place before, maybe more than once?

The ironic thing is that before stepping on that scale to assess my efforts, I was feeling pretty good. I'd been energetic and uncharacteristically optimistic about life that week, and it felt amazing to prioritize my self-care. But none of that mattered anymore—my optimism came to a screeching halt when that digital readout slapped an *F* for "failure" on all my efforts.

How did I go from feeling great and enthused about my progress only to let a number tank my self-esteem? *Does muscle really weigh more than fat, and that's why I weighed more? Was I just fooling myself into thinking I was making progress? Why does this have to be so hard?*

After this epic letdown, I threw my hands up in frustration and waved a white flag of surrender to my cravings. I ate "all the things" for a couple of weeks. I mean, why not? *If I'm not losing weight, what's the point of trying so hard?*

And eat and eat *and* eat I did.

During the weeks following that weigh-in, I felt awful. Sick, in fact. It seems a sugar-soaked sedentary lifestyle has a way of doing that to a girl.

I was weary and wanted something different for myself, but my motivation was withered like a flower in the scorching sun. I couldn't muster up the gumption to try once more—until my curiosity got the best of me and I stepped on the scale again. The upward tick of additional pounds woke me up like a splash of ice water on a chilly day. I blinked hard, but the number didn't change.

I'm not sure why I was so shocked by the weight gain. I guess some part of me felt like my overeating would slip through the cracks, but shielding ourselves from the truth only delays our realization that the effects of our choices accumulate.

Reality knocked, and my resolve returned once again. The more I thought about all the things I was doing wrong and all the areas

I fell short, the more desperate I felt to course correct. I couldn't live like this anymore, so I went searching for yet another diet to solve my struggles.

As I searched online for "best weight loss plans," I stumbled across a collection of before and after pictures. I was glued to the screen. But the more I scrolled, the greater the chasm between where I was and where I wanted to go seemed to be.

The difference felt irreconcilable. But I didn't know what else to do. Dieting was a way of life. I was snapped out of my trance only when my phone signaled me that my battery needed to be recharged. My spirit did too. I picked a diet and decided to start the very next day. *No, Monday.* I had so far to go, I didn't have the energy to begin now.

What a crummy way to start a new venture, don't you agree? I find it fascinating that we often stop at nothing to make sure our loved ones have everything they need to be successful, but meanwhile, we let ourselves begin from a place of deficit.

Thankful in All Circumstances

We all love to root for the underdog when we're on the sidelines, but starting behind the pack is a competitor's worst nightmare. Now, I'm about as competitive as a sloth, but I know what it's like to start from behind in dieting.

When we begin our umpteenth diet thinking about all we're not—forgetting our strength, overlooking our progress, blind to the blessings in front of us—that is starting from a place of deficit. Our eyes are locked on what we don't have in hopes that our discontentment will finally motivate us to change.

But starting from a place of negativity just breeds—you guessed it—more negativity. And that, my sis, is exactly the *opposite* of what we need when we begin a health journey.

Imagine how different it would feel to *cheer* yourself on to success rather than trying to be a drill sergeant. You'd feel encouraged and energized to keep going.

Let's remember how the Word of God instructs us to "give thanks in all circumstances" (1 Thess. 5:18), to praise the Lord and "forget not all his benefits" (Ps. 103:2), and to trust that "he who began a good work in [us] will bring it to completion" (Phil. 1:6).

So, what does it look like to exchange a diet-induced deficit for heavenly focused thankfulness for our bodies? We do it by meditating on all we *do* have and all we *are*. Now, this takes practice, and we'll look at how to get into a gratitude habit, but let's start by imagining what would happen if we were thankful in all circumstances.

When we are grateful instead of grumbling, we probably won't spend hours obsessing over the size of our thighs or squeezing our belly every time we pass a mirror. Rather, we'd celebrate how our legs let us keep up with our kids or our hands help us take care of older loved ones. If we're remembering God's benefits, meditating on all he has given us and thanking him for what he has done, we'll have less space to dwell on what we think we don't have. Instead, we'll praise the Lord for his provision. Are our pantry and refrigerator stocked with food? Then we can marvel at how we *get* to choose what we want to eat while others aren't so fortunate.

When you fix your eyes on the blessings in your life, you replace those perceived or exaggerated deficiencies with a knowledge of who God is and what he has already done for you. This shortens that daunting chasm between you and your goals, and you begin to see that you're not as far away from where you want to go as you thought you were.

The Ripple Effect of Gratitude

In the weeks leading up to Thanksgiving, social media feeds are plastered with reminders to celebrate what God has blessed us with. And the list is truly endless. When our eyes are on the hunt for blessings and benefits, they're not hard to find. Even in the most dire circumstances, a Christian whose life is secured in eternity can find something to praise the Lord for. Imagine gratitude as a heavenly spotlight that will shine even into your food struggles. The radiance of the light directs your eyes to the good things God has blessed you with, so much so you even forget about the "bad."

And that's the truth about focus. Negative thoughts lead to negative feelings, and that discomfort can land you smack-dab in the middle of a food fest. After all, when life is hard and nothing seems to be going your way, food is there to soothe your soul.

Have you ever noticed that eating can serve as an escape from mental mayhem? The negativity we steep ourselves in can be so painful and self-deprecating we may eat to escape our own internal dialogue. Which, as you may have guessed, can give us one more reason to beat ourselves up.

But *what if.*

What if thankfulness and gratitude reigned freely, and struggles were met with reminders of God's grace and mercy?

What if the downward spiral could be reversed and start to move you up, up, up?

What if you could stop working against yourself and watch your struggle become strength in his hands?

That's the power of gratitude. Gratitude lights your path to food freedom by training your mind to look for the good that happens each and every day. When you are encouraged, your motivation will remain strong and you'll keep showing up because this once arduous experience is now joy-filled.

Imagine waking up in the morning and, rather than ruminating on yesterday's struggles by replaying how you ate more than you planned, you open your eyes to the goodness of God. You pray, "God, I'm amazed at how you have provided for me. I have food to eat and a body that allows me to experience life—help me to honor you in my choices."

When it's time for breakfast, you don't force yourself to eat something prescribed by your latest diet (or rebel against those suggestions) but choose to fuel your body thoughtfully because, well, you're grateful for it. You consider what you'd like to eat and how you'd like to feel. That's a winning combination.

You get dressed and instead of spending fifteen minutes debating with yourself about your "trouble spots," you talk to the Lord about your struggles and trust he hears you: "Lord, you are the Potter and I am the clay. Help me not to despise what you have made. Thank you that I have so many clothes to choose from. I pray for those who are less fortunate."

As God shifts your thoughts to gratitude, you remember that your body allows you to do a lot of pretty amazing things.

Your internal environment is changing from hostile to helpful. Peace is beginning to reside in your heart and mind, and it soothes your soul. The more you talk to God, the more your desire to eat for comfort and escape diminishes.

Gratitude is the first step in this transformation because it aligns your thinking with biblical truth: You are *chosen*. Jesus died for you knowing all of your choices, and they didn't shake his adoration of you one bit. Let your imperfections remind you of his never-ending love. You are *fearfully and wonderfully made*. God formed you for a purpose, inside and out. When you see "problem areas," stretch yourself to celebrate that each is part of the package God made called *you*.

As you work your gratitude muscles, they'll become stronger, and you'll start to notice the good stuff much more easily. The less time you spend feeling in a funk, the less of a hold emotional eating will have on you. It all starts with where you look.

Looking up is the way out.

HABIT 1: GROW IN GRATITUDE

Each chapter of *Fully Nourished* introduces a new habit (or two to choose from). We'll walk through what it is, how it works, and how you practice it in a way that actually works in real life. Each habit is easy and doable, but don't let that fool you. When practiced consistently, they create lasting change. Over time, they'll become second nature, freeing up your energy to focus on the next grace-filled step. See how that works? (We'll take a deeper dive into how habits work in chapter 5.)

Your habit in this first chapter is to Grow in Gratitude, a practice that will exercise your mind and train your focus to be one that breathes *life* into your soul. To get started, you'll pick a time of day you'd like to write down or ponder what you are grateful for.

To make it stick, pair this new practice with something you're already doing. Habits are easiest to establish when anchored to another existing habit. For example, if you have a regular Bible study time, then completing your list before or after your study would be a natural segue. If you're already pretty strapped for time in the morning, then you could use your commute as a time to verbalize gratitude or create a talk-to-text list in a notes app. Other cues could be sitting down to breakfast, walking the dog, taking your lunch break, or putting kids to bed.

Once you have a time and anchor, think about how you'll *remind* yourself to Grow in Gratitude. Reminders are important because they turn ideas into actions, and actions are where your food freedom begins to blossom. Good reminders are placing a sticky note where you plan to complete your habit (it can be blank), setting an alarm on your phone, or putting a gratitude journal where you will see it when you need it.

The final step is to decide how many list items you want and what you would like to focus on.

Deciding "how many" comes down to picking a number that will stretch you without making this habit too hard. I recommend starting with ten, which should be enough to make you work a bit—you've got to *think* about what to write, and you'll probably need to start paying more attention throughout the day to get some ideas. However, if ten makes you want to shut this book and give up, pick a different number that makes you nod your head in agreement with your decision.

If you've done gratitude lists in the past, you probably thanked the Lord for your family, friends, and home. You applauded God for his faithfulness, provision, and unconditional love, and the world started to look a little bit brighter. But now you find yourself stepping into a new kind of journey—a faith-first approach to food freedom, where you're going to make peace with food and find joy in your body. So . . . why not start there?

If you're up for a challenge (and I really hope you are), focus half of your gratitude list on food and your body. This will start to center your attention on what God sees and begin to loosen those judgments you've held for a long time. Need a few ideas to get started? Try thanking God for things like these:

Taste buds that let you enjoy your favorite flavors.

A body that can move, rest, and heal.

Your ability to enjoy meals with people you love.

The smell of fresh coffee or a warm bowl of soup.

A heart that pumps without you even thinking about it.

Feet that follow the path God sets before you.

A voice to sing and hands to lift in praise.

These may seem simple, but they are sacred. Gratitude starts small and grows strong—just like your journey toward freedom.

Food gratitude can also be shown as thankfulness for having access to amounts of food that would make a large percentage of the world gasp in awe. Even if you're strapped for funds, your fridge probably has the essentials, and there is likely more than one type of cereal in your pantry. While food may feel like the enemy some days, having the option *to* overeat is a luxury.

Then there's gratitude for the way food tickles your senses. God could have made you to exist on air alone (and I've even wished for it), but in his goodness, he provides a beautiful variety of tastes and smells to enjoy. And food doesn't just taste good—food is *life*. Your genius Creator made food to nourish and fuel you so that you can do the things you love to do.

Your body is even more miraculous! While you may pinch and prod those "problem areas," I bet if you take some time to challenge those old ideas, you'll uncover the essence of praise. Your body is a marvel of God's goodness and can be an endless source of inspiration to honor him.

The belly that draws your attention when you pass a full-length mirror is the one that can take even the most unhealthy food and turn it into something that can keep you alive, without any of your help. The thighs that make jeans-shopping an annoyance belong to the same legs that carry you to your niece's dance recital, to the church auditorium to praise God, and to the bedside of an ailing loved one who needs your encouragement and prayer.

Think about your eyes, your ears, or your sense of touch. The way that bodies work is out of this world—and choosing to appreciate what God has given you will get you out of a body image funk faster than wiggling into some Spanx.

To sharpen your body-gratitude skills, I suggest going on YouTube and watching a few videos such as "How do my eyes work?" or "What happens to food when I eat it?" (I prefer kids' videos because they focus on wonder rather than bogging me down with hard-to-understand details.) Or head to the children's section at your local library, grab a few biology books, and find a cozy spot to flip through the pages.

Then use those awe-inspiring facts to combat negative body chatter. Over time, your automatic responses will begin to support your efforts to care for your body like it matters rather than judging it for something God doesn't even worry about.

PERSONALIZE YOUR HABIT

Now that you know what the outline of your new habit will be, it's time to move it from your brain into your heart and hands. The goal is to find a routine that works for *you*. You won't find a list of rules about what you *should* or *shouldn't* do here but a gathering of gentle guidelines that you'll use for a starting point.

A starting point is the place where you begin but not where you end up. While we'd all love to have the "perfect plan" right out of the gate, perfect rarely happens. This means, at some point, you'll pick a habit that *doesn't* work for you. No problem. Every experience offers insight. Even discovering that something does not work for you, or simply doesn't feel like a good fit, is valuable data. Every great scientist or world-changing inventor will tell you that knowing what doesn't work gets you one step closer to what does!

As I mentioned above, a good place to start to Grow in Gratitude is by writing down ten things you're grateful for each day—five general and five food- or body-specific (you can also adjust this habit by making it either easier or a bit more challenging). The key is that you feel about 80–90 percent confident you can practice your habit just about every day.

If you hesitate to commit, make your goal smaller. Right-sizing a habit so that you can be consistent is not failure—it's wisdom. Consistency is what you're aiming for because that's how habits take root. And when they do, they'll feel more natural, even on the hard days. Imagine having your healthy habits so ingrained you even do them on a bad day!

Remember to pick a specific time and place you'll Grow in Gratitude and consider how you're going to remind yourself to do what you intend. Here are a few examples to inspire you and remind you that there's no right or wrong here:

- I will write down ten things I am grateful for (five general/five body-specific) each day after I finish my

Bible study. To remind myself, I'll place a sticky note on my desk.

- I will use my commute to work to thank God for all he has done in my life. To remind myself, I will set an alarm on my phone. Then, I would also like to read some books on the amazing human body with my daughter.
- I will write down five things I am grateful for each day before I go to bed. To remind myself, I will put a notepad and pen on my bedside table.

The sky's the limit here! Pray and be inspired by the Holy Spirit to use this habit in a way that brings life to your heart and mind. Then practice this habit for the next week (or longer, if you want to take time to really let it sink in).

If you haven't done so yet, be sure to print out your free habit tracker and follow along with the included Scripture writing journal to keep your new habit and Jesus-first focus front and center. When you're ready, you'll move on to the next chapter and the next new habit.

Gratitude in Action

It was the year of Laura's twentieth wedding anniversary, and she and her husband were planning a dream vacation to Hawaii to celebrate with her immediate family. Ever since Laura was a little girl, she had imagined herself reclining on the beach amid miles of breathtaking coastline, gazing at turquoise blue water and an endless horizon. It really would be a dream come true.

But now she was struggling to get excited about their plans. Hawaii meant shorts, tank tops, and bathing suits. She was starting to panic when we first spoke about this upcoming adventure that she was now beginning to dread. She also felt guilty and awful for wanting to cancel such an incredible event.

I asked Laura to share some of her concerns. What was she thinking, and how were those thoughts affecting her anxiety? You see, while emotions can pop in uninvited, it is our thoughts that either nurture them or negate them.

It turned out that Laura's mind was brimming with fears and worry regarding her weight and the urgency to lose some of it. It was all she could think about. She kept threatening to go on a diet but never got around to it; instead she found herself binge eating to calm her anxieties and give herself a break from her negative thoughts.

"I just can't let it go," she confessed. "I can't celebrate my twentieth anniversary like *this*."

"Like what?" I asked. Laura went on to rattle off a list of all her perceived flaws.

When she finally took a breath, I broke her momentum with a different thought. "What's going to be *good* about this trip?"

She paused and began to share about the beauty of the beach, the excitement of the celebration, and the memories she would make with her family. Her voice changed, and I could hear joy bubbling up from her heart.

"Those are good things, right?" I asked redundantly.

Laura agreed.

"What would happen if you thought about those things instead?"

She took a few moments to let the question sink in and then, by the power of the Holy Spirit, a light bulb went off in her mind.

"Wow, I never thought about shifting my focus to something else. I actually feel better already."

Laura committed to stop trying to "fix" herself, and we devised a plan where she would spend the weeks leading up to the trip planning all the fun they would have, praying for her family, and even shopping for a swimsuit that made her feel great. She didn't go on a diet or spend hours at the gym, but she did fuel herself well and move her body more so that she would be better prepared to enjoy the early morning hikes they had planned.

And then she had "the best vacation ever."

She enjoyed eating "like a normal person" because food was not the primary focus before or during her time away. She wasn't stressed out about her body, and when insecurities popped in, she quickly reminded herself that this trip wasn't about being perfect but being with her people. All because she dared to believe that true joy wasn't found in shrinking her body but in expanding her view of God's goodness.

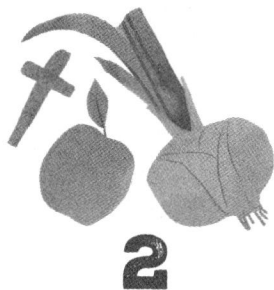

REJECT THE DIET MENTALITY

For freedom Christ has set us free; stand firm therefore,
and do not submit again to a yoke of slavery.

Galatians 5:1

It was half an hour past my bedtime; I should have been cozy in bed, fast asleep. But here I was, pacing around my kitchen—again—my attention fixated on the box of granola bars in the pantry.

I know I shouldn't eat one.

More pacing.

It's not on my plan.

I paced some more.

But it has chocolate chips!

I paused and then started pacing again.

Finally, the discomfort of indecision became too much—all my mental ping-pong felt like trying to help a toddler choose between the blue or the red truck. There was no end in sight, and I just wanted the decision to be over. So I tore open that shiny little wrapper and inhaled the granola bar. I hardly even tasted the chocolate, but I did feel somewhat relieved. I hid the wrapper in the trash and intended to move on.

But within a nanosecond, regret swooped in and snatched my momentary relief.

I hated this pattern, but I didn't know how to stop.

Frustration and disappointment welled up inside me. I felt like a volcano ready to erupt. I held back my lava tears and tried to bottle up my angst, but I was too upset to let this food failure go. You see, I'd started my day with such high hopes, convinced that today would be better.

I was going to:

Avoid the sugary creamer in my coffee.
Skip the cookie after lunch.
Drink only herbal tea during my afternoon slump.
Eat absolutely nothing after dinner.

Hour by hour, minute by minute, and bite by bite, I broke every one of those promises. Promises I'd made to myself, hoping I'd actually follow through this time but knowing I probably wouldn't.

It hurts to lose trust in yourself.

The sad thing is, I lived a high standard of always keeping the promises I made to other people, and I valued integrity. But I never considered the impact of letting myself down. It was depressing, and my self-talk wouldn't let me forget about those empty guarantees. By the time I entered my staring contest with that granola bar, I'd already spent hours ruminating on everything the enemy wanted me to believe.

I've already blown it.
It's too late to make a different choice.
I might as well eat the granola bar and try to do better tomorrow.

I was stuck, and I couldn't see a way out. Maybe you feel that way too.

How We Get Stuck

"You can't park here," I told my husband, pointing to the "No Parking" sign ten feet away and the bright yellow stripe on the curb warning us not to leave our vehicle there.

But he insisted. He only had a few boxes to unload, and I would stay in the car. It only took him a couple minutes to move those boxes, but it felt like an eternity as I sat restlessly, feeling guilty and waiting for the parking police to haul me off to jail.

I've always been a rule follower. Following the rules makes me feel protected, like I've done everything I can do to make others happy with me. Deviating from what I'm "supposed" to do leaves me feeling exposed and ashamed.

Thankfully, it's pretty easy to avoid parking in the wrong spot. My real problem was the endless list of diet rules I had to follow. Initially, all those rules felt comforting; I felt safe knowing what I could and couldn't do.

The concept of structure feels like freedom—until it becomes a jail.

The truth is, I wasn't able to keep following all the diet rules for long. I broke those laws every single day. But it wasn't the parking police who came for me. It was my internal Diet Dictator who locked me up.

Do it "right" or don't do it at all, my Diet Dictator demanded. So I handed over the remaining threads of hope I held. That's the nature of all-or-nothing thinking: It shines such a blinding spotlight on even the most insignificant imperfections that our brains begin to believe the only logical solution is to give up.

The last diet book you picked up likely lives in this All-or-Nothing Land, telling you to measure, weigh, classify, and count every bite you eat. Follow the formula and you'll be successful. The problem is, there are so many rules to follow it's impossible to keep them all. And maybe that's the point—many diet programs are structured to create dependency, not freedom. When you fail, they profit. Meanwhile, you feel guilty all the time, and the program makes it clear that any lack of success is entirely your fault. It's no wonder your sense of worth starts to get tangled up in the process.

Do you see how your value is attaching itself to your eating habits, and so every bite starts to feel like an act of either moral excellence or moral failure? The stakes are high, and the pressure to perform is intense.

Now, if there were no Diet Dictator to make you feel like a major failure, perhaps you'd move on after a less-than-ideal eating decision. But this internal perfectionistic tyrant won't let you. All-or-nothing thinking ambushes your brain, clouds your common sense, and convinces you to throw caution to the wind. You rationalize that since today will be the last day you'll ever eat Oreos, you've got to eat them ALL. Before the "nothing."

I want you to know that you're not alone. This pattern is so common—and so predictable—it can be boiled down to a series of well-worn steps.

Step 1: You start out the day with the best of intentions.
   Today is the day you're going to nail your eating and say no to every temptation that comes your way!

Step 2: Your intentions are challenged by an unexpected treat ("Oops, I ate so fast, I hardly tasted it!") or the desperate need for an escape ("I just need a break—now!").

Step 3: Feelings of failure and regret well up in your heart and mind. You feel terrible about your eating mistake and can't stop thinking about how disappointed you are in yourself.

Step 4: You answer your slip with the promise that you'll eat better—no, perfect—tomorrow.

Step 5: Those well-intentioned promises of perfect eating ramp up your fear of restriction, plopping you right into Last Supper Eating—when you eat like it's your last chance, before everything is off-limits tomorrow.

But this is not an addiction to food; it's a reaction to restriction. Can you imagine how different things would look if you stopped yourself at any one of these steps? It's not because you lack willpower. It's not even *about* willpower. No, this entire predicament was all spurred on by the Diet Dictator's directive to keep on restricting.

Did you catch that? You, an imperfect human, are expecting yourself to be able to eat perfectly through sheer willpower alone. Why? Because just about every diet book tells us that limiting the foods we love is the magic bullet that will fix our lack of self-control. Yet the backlash of such restrictions only increases our desire to eat.

And yet it's still scary to let those rules go.

What If You Never Stop Eating?

Are you afraid to break up with the Diet Dictator? I was! Maybe when you imagine a life without the "all" of following a diet, you worry that you'll never break free from the chaos of out of control eating. But as we've seen, it's the Diet Dictator that hijacks your brain and handcuffs your logical thinking.

Think about this: You don't let all-or-nothing thinking dominate other areas of your life. If you're going to be ten minutes late for church, you don't usually skip church, do you? No; you go because you value the remaining time you'll have, and you know it will make a difference in your life.

If you yell at your kids, do you throw in the towel on parenting? No way! You evaluate the trigger, apologize, and try to do better next time because your relationship is worth the effort.

Yet when it comes to your eating, do you often let a slip quickly become a slide, like I did? While it may seem illogical, you have pretty good reasons for doing this, even if they live in the worst-case scenario part of your brain.

You tell yourself, *If I don't have a diet to follow . . .*

I won't have a reason to say no to all those fattening foods.
I'll gain more weight trying to figure this out on my own.
I'll just keep eating because I'll have no reason to stop.

Those fears feel really real because the Diet Dictator has convinced you that your eating is something you must have total control over, and if you can only find the "right" diet, you'll suddenly have more self-control and will finally be able to take charge of your eating habits. That's a heavy burden to carry, and it's one you were never meant to bear on your own.

Yes, we can bring even our "What should I eat?" questions to the Lord.

It can be hard to let God in. You may be afraid that you've already disappointed him. Or you feel like you're the one who got yourself in this predicament, so you're the one who needs to get yourself out. It can also be scary to hand your weight loss over to God and let him decide what you should weigh. After all, what if God doesn't care how you look in a swimsuit?

It's okay to wrestle with these questions. Your heavenly Father knows your struggles. He sees the worries that play like a movie in your mind. And he doesn't condemn or shame you. God's desire is to calm your anxiety with his perfect love and cover your weaknesses with his grace.

Yet God's grace may feel scary too.

If you fear "grace" in your eating, it's probably because you misinterpret what it looks like. You may be mistaking grace for license. You imagine you'll never stop eating if there's no need to tally every bite, and you'll never consume a stalk of broccoli again. But God's grace isn't an excuse to eat everything in sight. It isn't a free pass to indulge every last craving. No, God's grace holds a higher standard—a measurement of your heart rather than your behavior.

Your heavenly Father cares about what you *love* more than what you do.

Grace makes it possible for you to please God, even if you're stuck in an emotional eating battle. Your relationship with him is more important than your performance. Any sequence of events, as frustrating as they may be, that ends with you loving Jesus more can be counted as a win.

When you ask the Lord for help, regardless of what happened two hours or two bites ago, you practice turning to him in times of need and strengthen your walk with him. When you ask for forgiveness and celebrate that Jesus's blood has covered every struggle, you become even more proficient in praising him and magnifying his name. And when you break the power of the Diet Dictator, you free yourself to tune in to God's still, small voice that will gently guide your eating choices.

You can't fail when you end up in God's arms, regardless of the path it took to get you there. Don't let the enemy or your perfectionistic tendencies tell you otherwise.

Only God Is Perfect

You know that moment when we realize our kids *are* actually absorbing what we say?

My moment came at our kitchen table, which held more craft supplies than dinner plates. My daughter, just shy of two, sat admiring her masterpiece: Random pompoms dripping with glue, a smattering of buttons, and dried pasta adorned her once ordinary sheet of construction paper. "Perfect!" she announced, chin up and shoulders high. Her enthusiasm was adorable, and I celebrated how she saw her creation as a Picasso.

But that word, that one that has caused you and me so much angst and pain—*perfect*—began to slip into her conversation. She folded a towel into jumbled, uneven squares: "Perfect!" She attempted a somersault, raised her short little arms: "Perfect!" And she even brushed her hair, staring into her eyes in the mirror, and whispered to herself, "Perfect."

While she did not understand the full weight of the word, my recovering perfectionist brain went on high alert. Perfectionism would not steal her joy like it had mine.

I explained to her that humans could never be perfect in the way God required, and our humanness was nothing to be ashamed of because only Jesus is perfect. We agreed to ban the word *perfect* from our home, and when it slipped out, as it often did, we reminded ourselves that "Only God is perfect."

It was a fun game where she got to correct her mama—a lot.

As much as you and I would love to be flawless, it'll never happen this side of heaven. It isn't available to us. To allow our human state to keep us up at night is fruitless and exhausting.

Your best response to those reminders of reality is not to stay stuck but to use the realization as an opportunity to glorify God. Have a food slip? Repent if needed, move on, and celebrate that only God is perfect. He saved you despite your struggles. Your food slips and slides don't shake his adoration. Let the joy of God's unconditional love fill your heart and seep out of your mouth because this is a message the world needs to hear.

So, how do you change your habits if you're not "all in" on eating well? The truth is, God's economy works incredibly different from our world's, and all he asks for is a "little," given with your full heart.

The Power in a "Little"

I'm not a gardener, but I married a man with a green thumb. The planting season is an exciting one as my husband and daughter gather new packets of seeds on the patio table. Some look familiar to me, such as green peppers, tomatoes, and strawberries. And even though I've seen strawberry seeds on the outside of that delicious fruit, it still amazes me to see how God made our food so brilliantly reproducible.

I also find it incredible how that little bag of hard-to-spot strawberry seeds costs more than a quart of fresh Florida berries. Seems crazy, right? Except when you know the potential of a seed. That near-invisible speck has the internal possibility to birth buckets of strawberries. *If* it is planted.

I bet you're wondering what this analogy has to do with food freedom. Well, the reality is that we find ourselves planting seeds all the time. Seeds are our thoughts, behaviors, and actions that grow into the framework of our lives.

If you're planting seeds of doubt and fear, your mind is probably pretty anxious. If you're planting seeds of unrealistic expectations and perfectionism, you're probably pretty stressed out. And if you're planting seeds of dietary restriction followed by a lack of restraint, you probably feel at the mercy of your cravings.

But what if you started planting a new kind of seed? The kind of seed that would produce the kind of relationship with food you longed for?

A Seed of Self-Control.

HABIT 2: SOWING SEEDS OF SELF-CONTROL

Your habit this chapter is Sowing Seeds of Self-Control, a daily practice where you'll surrender to the Lord "bite-size" seeds—food or otherwise. These are tiny, faith-filled actions that will build hope in your ability to change as you successfully make tiny offerings to God, day by day.

A seed is small but mighty. The object sown in the soil is tiny compared to the full-grown plant that hopefully will emerge. In the realm of behavior change, you're also aiming for small but mighty action steps. Steps that are so simple you're confident you can do them consistently while also being valuable enough that you *want* to.

Sowing Seeds of Self-Control can take on many forms because your relationship with food can be improved through a variety of habits. From what you think about to taking an after-work walk, seeds that improve your overall health and happiness will have a welcome ripple effect on how you eat.

Your tiny seed could be swapping out one soda a day for water or "tithing bites" by leaving three bites of food on your dinner plate. These are doable actions but still require a small sacrifice on your part so that you have the opportunity to rely on the Lord for his strength. But, unlike a diet, you'll make sure the action is easy enough for you to be consistently successful.

The "go big or go home" methods of dietary improvements have not worked for us in the past because they were based on self-effort. It's time to step out in faith and trust that God can do a lot with our little.

And if we're honest, our "little" *is* a lot because we've held on to our relationship with food with tight fists for quite a while. Letting our heavenly Father into our eating is far more productive than passing on a piece of chocolate cake all while lusting for it in our hearts.

Today, your transformation is coming from the inside out!

To get started, you'll want to identify the first seed you'd like to plant. Then you can begin to map out the details of your habit practice. Please note: You may not pick the perfect seed to start, and that's okay. Only God is perfect, remember? The goal is not mastery but experimentation and consistency. So have fun with it!

Let me give you a few examples to get started. This list is designed to inspire you and is not a to-do list. You'll find several ideas to pull from, but the sky's the limit. Follow the leading of the Holy Spirit within you and be led by your peace. If leaving three bites behind makes you want to run for the hills or stirs up old, unhelpful patterns—honor those feelings.

- Go for a ten-minute walk after dinner.
- Swap out your afternoon sweet with some fruit and cheese.
- Put a small amount of food back when serving yourself dinner.

- "Fast" for ten minutes during a challenging eating window.
- Add veggies to your dinner.
- Pray a short prayer every time you open the fridge.
- Swap your most pervasive negative thought for a new Scripture-inspired one.
- "Tithe bites" by leaving three bites behind at dinner.
- Listen to praise music or a sermon instead of the news when you get home from work.
- Say "no thanks" to second helpings at meals and wait twenty minutes before deciding if you need to eat more.
- Determine to reset after an eating slip before it turns into a slide.

Each of these can be done from a place of sacrifice to the Lord *or* be done mindlessly. As you choose which seed to sow, be sure to *purposefully* plant it. Avoid the diet mindset where the habit becomes all about you and your eating; instead, make it about you and the Lord.

Let's say you choose to go for a ten-minute walk after dinner. Ask the Lord to give you the fortitude to step outside when you really would rather veg out on the sofa. On the walk, thank God for the ability to move your body and for the creation you see as you're outside. Then, when you get home, praise him for being faithful to you!

Practically speaking, this habit also has a lovely ripple effect beyond those ten minutes. Walking gets you out of the habit of nibbling while you clean up after dinner. Moving your body after eating means you won't want to eat too much, and physical activity is great for regulating your blood sugar after your meal. Now you'll arrive home in a better headspace and probably sleep better too!

Can you see how that's a seed that grows? Every tiny, healthy habit seed does this, whether you can pinpoint it or not.

PERSONALIZE YOUR HABIT

Are you ready to pick your starting point? Decide on a small seed you feel 80–90 percent confident you can sow just about every day. If you're wavering on your ability to be consistent, make your seed easier. It's far better to choose a seed you can and will plant because even the smallest seeds can take root and produce fruit.

Then decide on a time and place you'll sow a Seed of Self-Control and consider how you're going to remind yourself to do what you intend. Here are a few examples to inspire you and remind you that there's no right or wrong here:

I will take an apple and nut butter to work for my afternoon snack (instead of hitting up the vending machine). I will prepare my snacks on the weekend and leave my cash in the car, so I'm not tempted to purchase additional snacks.

When I hear negative body chatter, I will replace those thoughts with this truth from God's Word: The Lord made me, and I am his. He rejoices over me with singing (Zeph. 3:17). To remind myself, I will write this truth on 3×5 cards and put one on my mirror and one in my closet. I'll also change the screensaver on my phone.

I will tithe some bites and put a small scoop of food back when I serve myself dinner. To remind myself, I will put a vase with flowers on the table.

There are so many possibilities to play with and, with time and practice, you'll find a seed that inspires and transforms you!

Practice this habit for the next week (or longer, if you want to take time to really let it sink in). Be sure to use your habit tracker and follow along with the included Scripture writing journal to keep your new habit and Jesus-first focus front and center.

Planting Seeds in Any Weather

I'd already "blown" my diet, and here I was again. My internal Diet Dictator was enticing me to give up, and I found myself wearing a path between the pantry and the refrigerator. I opened the fridge, hoping I'd overlooked some leftover goodies, but nothing sweet magically appeared there. I scoured the cupboards, searching for the ingredients to whip up brownies. But alas, I'd thrown out the cocoa powder after my last kitchen raid. Nevertheless, the truth was I didn't have eggs either, or the patience to wait for a baked treat.

The indecision wore me down, and I finally broke under the pressure. I decided to eat just to shut up the chatter in my mind. So I ate a bowl of cereal. I felt hopeless and defeated, and the pattern I'd lived throughout the last decade continued—I'd answer my perceived failure with more food while I promised myself that tomorrow would be different.

That moment in the downward spiral felt irrevocable. It was a pattern I'd practiced more times than I could count, and I was persuaded I could never break free.

But then something happened that I will never forget.

God, in his great mercy, whispered into my heart, *You can stop. No, I can't!* I insisted. *The damage has already been done.*

Much to my surprise, for what felt like the first time in my life, logic and reason entered my mind. The living and active Word of God I had consumed and the verses that echoed food freedom came to life within me. *Eating more is not going to help*, I thought, with a hint of conviction. *Step away, find something else to do. Take this as a win.*

A win?! my worn-out diet brain protested. *You've got to be kidding me—your eating has failure written all over it. You might as well have another bowl of cereal.*

Condemnation and the Word of God went to war in my heart and mind, but God won.

I won.

I walked away, did something else, and celebrated it as a success. And you know what? It felt really, really good. The thing that surprised me the most was that I ate so much less that day than if I'd gone down that old, dusty Binge Boulevard. A light went off in my mind, and I started to see the power of God's grace. I was forgiven, I had a fresh start, and I wanted to do better.

The same goes for you, sis. When you embrace that seeds grow, you can begin to plant seeds that will produce the crop you desire to harvest.

And it all starts with Sowing Seeds of Self-Control.

3

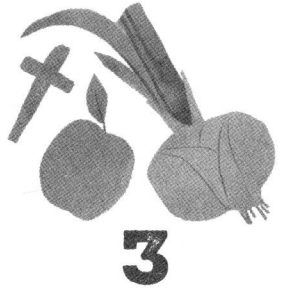

ALIGN YOUR BODY IMAGE
WITH GOD'S WORD

My frame was not hidden from you, when I was being made in secret, intricately woven in the depths of the earth.

Psalm 139:15

It's going to be fun, I tried to assure myself. *People just want to see you, and nobody cares about your weight.*

My internal words fell on deaf ears. My self-conscious self wasn't having it—there was no way I was going to that birthday party. I knew I'd be with friends I hadn't seen in a while, and, well, I didn't want them to see me. Not like "this."

The part of me that valued spending time with loved ones battled the part of me that affixed my worth and value to my appearance. I longed to hug my teenage Bible study bestie, but I was too embarrassed for her to see how I'd "let myself go."

And, of course, there would be food. Lots of it. *What does a girl who's gained weight eat?* I wondered. *If I eat the salad, everyone will probably wonder how I gained weight, but if I have some birthday cake, they'll know how I did.*

Why couldn't I just get dressed and go?

Why did I believe others would scrutinize my body like I did?

Why did I miss that celebration?

My stomach still churns when I think about all the special events I avoided because of how I felt in my own skin. Places and people I longed to see, all missed, while I sat at home and mourned and . . . ate.

It took me a while to unravel the vicious cycle I'd created. The one where my isolation and negative body chatter separated me from the experiences that would make me feel "full," no chocolate required.

God wired us to need one another, but I was so focused on myself I didn't see it. It's probably because I never asked the Lord into my struggle; I only pleaded for him to help me stop overeating. I guess I didn't think God would understand and, if I'm honest, I was afraid he'd leave me unhappy in my skin forever. With so many major problems in the world, why would God care about how my jeans fit or how many events require a bathing suit here in sunny Florida?

Self-isolated from biblical wisdom, I kept operating in the same broken mindset: "If I can only lose weight, *then* I'll live the life I was meant to, and *then* I can walk confidently into what God has called me to do!"

But I was adding steps to God's plan. Like a Pharisee, I was trying to change only the outside, forgetting that I could never add to the finished work of Jesus Christ on the cross. When God wants to use someone, he will. The Bible doesn't speak about any physical prerequisites, including our poundage, to be used for his purposes. It was my self-doubt holding me back, and it wasn't God who told me I was fat.

Where Lies Begin

I grew up in the '90s—an era of teased hair, SnackWell's fat-free cookies, and supermodels. While some girls dreamed of becoming doctors, I wanted to be a model. I spent hours flipping through fashion magazines, even holding up photos of "perfect" women while scanning my own reflection for flaws.

That was more than a few years ago, and the rip current has only taken us further away from what the Bible says is important. Today, we can compare ourselves to endless filtered, curated images of influencers with just a scroll. We're constantly submerged in artificial perfection and messages that whisper, "You're not enough."

But thin hasn't always been in. Throughout history, especially in times when food was scarce, a fuller figure signaled wealth and fertility. In fact, it wasn't until the early 1900s that fashion began favoring thinner frames—not because they were "better" but because they made it easier to drape fabric and design patterns. It was about function, not beauty. Just like jockeys are small so that horses are fast and basketball players are tall so they can be closer to the hoop, fashion chooses functional frames too.

Somewhere along the way, we took cultural ideals to heart and began chasing what fashion and the world deemed desirable— ignoring what God had already called good. As Christians, we can recognize the contrast. Yet the world's voice is loud and the cultural current is strong. Even the best-intentioned believers can get swept up in the tide, slowly losing sight of God's truth and wading into discontentment—especially when it comes to our bodies.

But what's even more difficult? When the source of negative body baggage is much, much closer. Sometimes the loudest voices aren't on a magazine or a screen—they come from the people closest to us.

For me, that moment came as a young girl at my best friend's house, when a spur-of-the-moment remark made me feel like my body wasn't quite right. I don't think the comment was meant to wound, but it struck deep. From that day on, I began to see myself through a different lens—a critical one.

You have your own story too, I'm certain. One where someone planted a seed of inadequacy into the soil of your heart. And no matter what the actual words were, you heard and felt "I'm not okay." Then, with time and cultural cultivation, that thought burrowed roots of inadequacy and grew a self-image that has haunted you ever since. Now the lies feel too deeply rooted to pluck out. For any human, that is.

But God can do what we never thought was possible.

The Day I Put My Foot Down

I sat on the edge of the sofa with my head buried in my hands. Though my eyes were closed, I could see the last twenty years of my life pass through my mind like a memorial slideshow. Each snapshot was the same . . . me agonizing over my weight and obsessing over my appearance, desperate for accolades from others. I saw myself go from a hopeful preteen to a weary thirtysomething in a downward spiral accelerated by each and every diet I tried. Regret welled up in my belly and planted itself in my throat. I had nothing left to give. Nothing left to do.

I was empty.

As painful as it is to feel like we've wasted years, it's also a relief to realize we don't have the power to solve our own problems. I mean, what else could I do? I'd tried dozens of programs, seen dietitians and therapists, and even spent six weeks at an eating disorder treatment center. But all those failed attempts made me feel even more broken.

Maybe too broken to fix.

"God," I prayed, "I've got nothing left to give. I can't fight this anymore. I can't live like this anymore. I'm tired of hating myself. I'm tired of running to food. I don't want to think about *me*, I want to think about *you*."

I suspect it took all those years to loosen my controlling grip, but oh, how I wish that last effort had been my first. Because in that moment, something changed. By a power not my own, I stood up, looked up, and put my foot down, declaring a holy refusal to stay stuck in that miserable place.

That day, I realized that changing my body wouldn't fix my discontented heart or critical vision. I needed to start *believing* what God's Word said about me—that he examined my heart, not my waistline. That I was created on purpose, for a purpose. And that his love wasn't waiting until I lost ten pounds—it was already mine. And I did believe it.

Not because I felt like it.

Not because I suddenly loved my body.

But because I was done living in shame.

The negative self-talk still showed up. But I stopped entertaining it. I chose to respond like God's truth was *actually true*—because I was starting to believe it was.

And the more I leaned in to that truth by faith, the more I softened toward myself. My reflection began to shift—not because my jeans fit differently but because I finally saw myself through God's eyes. Joy welled up in my belly and planted a new song in my heart. I finally began experiencing the fullness that comes from soaking in God's unconditional love—and with that fullness, food began to lose its grip on me.

You may be pondering how you can finally put your foot down, flip the switch, and start feeling joyful in your own skin. You're weary from fighting against yourself but, if you're honest, you're a little nervous too.

If you're like me, you've wondered, *What if the Lord doesn't care about my weight as much as I do?* After all, appearance has never been a qualification for you to love others—why would it be for God? So, then, you feel a little guilty for even caring about something as superficial as your appearance.

You start to wonder what it would look like to let go of those long-held ideals. *If I accept where I am, am I just giving up? What happens to my goals?* It's confusing. Overwhelming. Sometimes even paralyzing. And this tug-of-war in your mind is the very thing that keeps you stuck—cycling through self-criticism, striving, and shame.

I was under the impression that I had to pick one or the other: to focus solely on inward beauty *or* feel happy in my own skin. And the assumption that these were two polarizing sides kept me stuck, trying to fight this battle on my own.

However, the Word of God doesn't say anywhere that it is sinful to feel beautiful. It's when we put our appearance before our relationship with God, our character, or loving others that things start to go haywire. Our confidence is to be in Christ, but a new haircut, manicure, or outfit can make a girl feel seriously great. Denying yourself these things until you reach a certain weight only does you a disservice.

Our God is the maker of lovely things. Everything he makes is wonderful. Including *you*.

So, how do you cultivate this perspective? You start by understanding what the Bible says about you and believing it by faith, until the seeds planted by the Word of God germinate in your heart and mind and change how you see yourself. As you practice the habits taught in this book and begin to treat yourself as one worthy of care, your self-perception will begin to heal and align with God's Word, whether the scale changes or not.

Three Godly Truths

When you start holding your beliefs up to God's truth, you may notice some of them haven't served you well at all. Feeling bad about your body has held you back more than you ever realized. It's not just about weight, inches, or even bathing suit shopping. It's about peace, joy, and quality of life. It's time to stop trading your happiness for a media-induced mirage and walk in the fullness God has for you!

These next three truths were *my lifeline* and turning point in my journey toward healing. I encourage you to make them yours too. Print out the companion cards included in your free download (or jot them down on a 3×5 card) and display them near your closet, on your bathroom mirror, and anywhere else you can think of plastering them.

Truth #1: You Were Crafted by God

For we are his workmanship, created in Christ Jesus for good works, which God prepared beforehand, that we should walk in them. (Eph. 2:10)

My dad is a gifted artist. He studies a blank canvas and sees unlimited potential. He adds a few "random" strokes of paint and, layer by layer, creates a masterpiece. Those of us watching from the outside can't fathom how each swipe of his brush fits into the whole, but the artist knows.

God created you thoughtfully and intentionally, purposing each brushstroke. And while you may wonder why you're the only one with red hair in your family, why you can play the piano effortlessly but can't balance your checkbook, or why you were born with the eyesight of a bat, it's not a cosmic accident. Each and every brushstroke of you is part of the Artist's creation and part of your purpose.

You are God's masterpiece.

Truth #2: Your Body Is a Marvel

I praise you, for I am fearfully and wonderfully made.
Wonderful are your works;
    my soul knows it very well. (Ps. 139:14)

Not only are you a masterpiece but you're also a marvel. While science has come a long way, not even the greatest scientific visionary could envision the intricacies of how God created you.

Imagine a mundane task you do every day, such as washing dishes or brushing your teeth. None of it would be possible without divine design. You know when the water is too hot or when you've grabbed the wrong flavor of toothpaste. It's not accidental, it's monumental. When you take the time to observe, celebrate, and meditate on the marvel of the gift God has given you in your body, you'll begin to soften toward yourself. And in that softening, you'll discover more to be grateful for than you ever imagined.

You are God's beautiful creation.

Truth #3: Beauty Is More Than Skin-Deep

But let your adorning be the hidden person of the heart with the imperishable beauty of a gentle and quiet spirit, which in God's sight is very precious. (1 Pet. 3:4)

We've been robbed by the worldly definition of beauty, which assumes that something or someone is only pleasant to the eye if it meets certain proportions or aesthetics. But it turns out that what draws us to a person, place, or thing is less about its appearance and more about how it makes us feel.

The beautiful sunset you enjoy on a summer evening is painted with strokes of vibrant hues. But what draws you back is not the shades of fuchsia and saffron but how those blankets of color make you *feel*.

Consider our Lord and Savior Jesus Christ. The Bible says Jesus was considered plain and did not have an appearance that would cause others to be attracted to him (Isa. 53:2). But those who longed for unconditional love and acceptance were drawn to him because he made them feel worthy of love. Even David, considered a man after God's own heart, didn't look the part of a king. To everyone's surprise, our Creator, in his wisdom, purposefully crafted David to challenge the ideals of those around him.

Beauty is not a moving target dictated by the finicky tastes of our culture but an attribute of one who reflects the love of Jesus— one who makes others feel seen, loved, heard, and understood.

You are God's reflection.

Whether or not you fully believe those three points yet, they are indeed true. That's important to note because it's the truth that sets you free (John 8:31–32). Take some time to challenge your beliefs and negative self-talk that have held you back. It can be scary to step away from what you've always known, and it's normal to feel attached to what's familiar, even if it's harmful. It's okay.

Take a deep breath; there's nothing you have to change right now. Listening—to your body, your emotions, and God's voice—is the first step to healing.

What Does Your Body Say to You?

We've spent some time exploring what *you* have to say about your body, but what does your body have to say to you? You likely have some strong opinions about what size and shape you "should" be, and you may also carry some hidden expectations about how your body should *feel*, both physically and emotionally.

Your body can tell you a lot about what's going on in your heart and mind. That's why our habit for this chapter is the Mind-Body Scan. You're going to take a few moments each day to see what's happening underneath the hood. This will put you in a great position as you move forward, giving you a sneak peek into your hunger and fullness signals as well as increasing your awareness of the thoughts and feelings that send you to the pantry. Then, as you progress through the book, you'll have a head start identifying your deeper needs, and you'll learn how to preemptively meet those needs before they feel too challenging to navigate.

For too long, far too many of us have seen our bodies as a burden. We can rattle off a laundry list of all the things we'd like to change, missing the blessing the Lord has given us.

Your physical being—the part of you that interacts with the world—is resilient and fragile at the same time. Your body can endure more than you realize but is more sensitive than you give it credit for. By consistently practicing the Mind-Body Scan and connecting with who God made you to be, you'll grow in grace and appreciation for yourself. This will empower you to live in an authentic way that can change the world around you!

Before we walk through how to practice this habit, let's take a look at the two major disconnects the Mind-Body Scan can help you begin to repair.

The Emotional Disconnect

Emotions are unpredictable and tricky to navigate, especially if you've never been taught how to manage their waves. Maybe as a kid you were told to stop crying when you were hurt, to push aside anger when things didn't go your way, or to feel embarrassed about your anxiety or fears. Or maybe the instruction to bypass your feelings was more subtle—you recognized your emotions influenced those around you, so you put on a happy face and buried your feelings to avoid causing distress to others.

Then you got older and life got more complicated. Your best friend moved across the country, you lost the scholarship you so desperately needed, or you found yourself struggling to fit in at college. You didn't know what to do with your feelings; they were so uncomfortable and awkward, and you found yourself eating to soothe yourself. Bite by bite, you drowned out your feelings until every unwelcome emotion started to feel like a call to eat.

The Physical Disconnect

Emotional disconnect isn't the only way we lose touch with our bodies. We also struggle to interpret our physical needs—especially after years of dieting.

While we all have our reasons for going on our first diet, the results for each of us were the same: We handed our autonomy about *what to eat, how much to eat,* and *when to eat* over to a plan or program. It was no longer about how hungry or full we were but whether or not the plan said it was time to eat. We ate seven almonds when we wanted twelve, and we ate an extra yogurt at

10:00 p.m. even though we weren't hungry, just because we still had some calories or points left. And it felt kind of good to transfer the responsibility of what to eat to someone or something else. But this only widened the disconnect we had with our bodies. With each diet, the chasm grew wider, making our "it's time to eat" and "it's time to stop eating" signals a language we could not understand.

If your body signals, both physical and emotional, feel messier than the tangle of cords found behind your television, you're not alone. The Mind-Body Scan will begin to reconnect you with what your body is saying both emotionally and physically and will pave the way for future habits.

❖ ❖ ❖ ❖ ❖

Before we delve into the how-tos of the Mind-Body Scan, it's essential to clarify what this habit is *not*. The Mind-Body Scan is not about fixing or altering anything. In fact, if you find yourself over-thinking, stuck in self-criticism, or trying to force yourself to feel differently, you won't reap the scan's full benefits. To gain insight, you've got to observe what is genuinely occurring within yourself, without imposing your preconceived ideas or expectations. Then as you move forward, you'll uncover the proper salve—self-care, prayer, or savory meal—to apply to your needs.

One final word of encouragement: If you've been tuning out these signals for a while, don't expect to grasp them right away. Truthfully, you may not even feel like you're doing the Mind-Body Scan correctly, and that's okay. Let me assure you that *by simply paying attention*, you're doing just fine.

Your one and only job is to listen to you.

HABIT 3: MIND-BODY SCAN

A Mind-Body Scan is a purposeful pause where you notice what is happening in your mind and how your body is feeling. It can take fifteen seconds or three minutes, depending on the goal and context. The best part about this exercise is that it can be done in a quiet, empty room or in the bleachers at a playoff game. All you need is you.

Here are the three simple steps to get started.

Step 1: Notice

Start at the top of your head and take note of how it feels. Is it tense or relaxed? Do you feel any sensations?

Slowly move down and notice your mind. Is it busy or calm? Do you feel anxious or peaceful? Are your thoughts running wild, or are you taking your thoughts captive?

Keep moving down. Are any emotions showing up in your body, creating a physical expression such as stress-induced tight shoulders or an anxiety-acquired bellyache?

Next, notice your current need for food. Do you feel a physical need or emotional craving to eat? (In your mouth? In your stomach?)

Continue scanning down, being aware of the bodily sensations you feel as well as how your emotional state may be affecting your body.

That's it. You've successfully done a Mind-Body Scan!

Step 2: Name

So, what do you do with your discoveries? You're going to name them. Naming is simply giving description to what you noticed so that you can state "Just the facts, ma'am" and avoid overthinking, overdramatizing, and overreacting (which often lead to overeating!).

Say, "I feel [fill in the blank]."

I feel tense, and my mind is racing.

I feel hungry in my throat but not in my belly.

I feel tired, and my mind is filled with thoughts of sugar, but I'm not hungry.

I feel anxious and jittery, and my shoulders are scrunched all the way up to my ears.

Step 3: Note

If you uncover anything notable in your naming, jot it down in a journal or in the notes app on your phone. If you don't notice anything, no worries. Just by being aware, you have communicated to yourself that what you feel *matters*.

In time, you'll start to notice patterns. You may find that you're more anxious than you realized or that your hunger signals feel different than you expected them to. You may discover that frustration makes you want to chew or your desire for chocolate and coffee at 3:00 p.m. is actually the call for a brain break.

Of course, you won't see all of this right away, so no pressure to solve an epic mystery. Simply note it. We'll circle back around to what you uncover in the next chapter.

PERSONALIZE YOUR HABIT

To make the Mind-Body Scan a sustainable habit, you'll want to anchor it to things you already do every day. This way you'll be sure to get into a memorable routine. Start by choosing one or two realistic and consistent times each day, such as waking up, going to bed, or eating a meal, where you can set aside a few moments to pause and reflect. Don't aim for perfect, just *present*.

Here are a few ways you could practice your Mind-Body Scan. Remember: More isn't better if more is too much. Keep it doable and sustainable to increase your chances of creating a long-term habit.

As soon as I wake up, I will do a Mind-Body Scan. To help me remember, I will change the tone of my alarm clock.

Before breakfast, I will do a Mind-Body Scan. To help me remember, I will put a sticky note on the table where I eat.

Before every meal, I will do a Mind-Body Scan. To help me remember, I will set an alarm on my phone near my normal mealtimes.

I also encourage you to use your scan as a quick check-in throughout the day. If you spend the next couple of weeks gathering information that reveals the thoughts, feelings, and emotions that complicate your relationship with food, it'll be one of the best investments you'll make along this journey.

Again, please don't stress about getting this "right." This is an intangible habit, and there's no measurement of a good or bad Mind-Body Scan. The mere act of paying attention is the win!

Changing What You See, Changing the World

Jenna knew the Lord had been calling her to the worship team for years, but she always talked herself out of stepping forward. She was terrified of standing in front of the entire congregation when she felt so uncomfortable in her body. The enemy whispered into her ear that everyone would be looking at her, judging her.

Yet Jenna loved to praise the Lord through music. She glowed from the inside out as she glorified his name, and she had a gift for leading others into his throne room through the power of praise. But her self-conscious self wasn't having it. She just couldn't get past her negative body image.

Until her beliefs were challenged in a most unexpected way.

After church on a Wednesday evening, Jenna was chatting with her friend Natalie about the pastor's message on the importance of prayer. Natalie expressed how she'd been longing to join the prayer team, but she hesitated because she felt self-conscious about her weight. She was frustrated by her lack of commitment to her health and her struggles with self-control and, therefore, felt disqualified to publicly pray for others.

Jenna couldn't believe what she was hearing. She'd always admired Natalie and saw her as a beautiful, godly woman. Like a mama bear defending her child from a schoolyard bully, Jenna refuted the lies that kept her friend stuck. Natalie *was* qualified because she loved Jesus, she was a daughter of the king, and the Holy Spirit resided in her.

Just . . . like . . . me . . .

That truth bomb dropped into Jenna's spirit, and her self-image began to shift. It started to become clear that it wasn't God who told her she was unqualified. That was a lie from the enemy. She got fired up, put her foot down, and made a decision to no longer stay stuck.

Putting your foot down isn't just about defiance—it's a declaration. A holy rebellion against the lies of the enemy.

Later that month, Jenna tried out the worship team, and something pretty unexpected and absolutely amazing began to happen. She felt a joy she'd never experienced before as she stepped into the calling God had for her life.

Obedience tastes amazing.

As her life became richer, she thought less about herself and less about food. Jenna grew in confidence as she grew closer to the Lord.

She and Natalie became two powerful forces for Jesus. No wonder Satan wanted to keep them sitting on the sidelines. Imagine what would happen if Christian women quit entertaining the constraints of worldly definitions of beauty, embraced what God said about them, and shined for Jesus?

The world would never be the same.

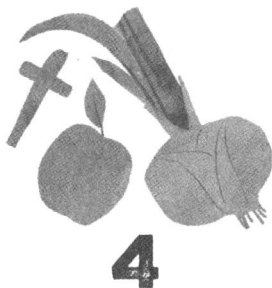

UNCOVER THE GOALS
THAT MOTIVATE YOU

*But seek first the kingdom of God and his righteousness,
and all these things will be added to you.*

Matthew 6:33

What if the reason you can't seem to stay motivated on an eating plan is because you're doing it for the wrong reasons? What would happen if you uncovered goals that *actually* motivate you, even on a hard day?

What would it feel like to pass on the second helping of pie, not because you have to and not because it has too much sugar but because skipping it aligns with who you see yourself as?

I'd been so "good" on my diet, nailing my portions, hitting my macro goals, and eating foods I didn't even like. I felt like I was finally gaining some traction (for the day, at least), but then I saw it: leftover cookie cake in the employee lounge. I just wanted to taste the icing, but then I saw a chocolate chunk too. So I cut just a small slice (I think you know where this is going). I ended up eating a massive piece of that cake, one sliver at a time, completely paranoid that a coworker would walk in and see me blowing my diet. I felt embarrassed and ashamed.

To make matters worse, I didn't even enjoy that cake.

Why would I say that I wanted to lose weight, pay significant money for a diet plan, invest the first half of my day into nailing the program, and then eat like I didn't care? This is the thought that puzzled me, diet after abandoned diet. I made pretty good choices in other areas of my life; maybe I didn't care about weight loss as much as I thought I did?

Have you ever contemplated the same thing, scratching your head at the inconsistencies and extremes of your eating habits?

You and I are not alone. Almost everyone is bombarded with the reasons we should want to be a certain size or shape—but is it possible they aren't *your* reasons? Maybe you have the insight and wisdom to realize that weight loss is never going to be the promised land you've been told it is. And the discomfort of saying no to a craving, enduring emotional turmoil, or eating fish for the third time in a week is just not worth the mirage of weight loss far in the distance.

Arrival fallacy is the belief that reaching a goal or end point will lead to long-term happiness. It's a false assumption that once you achieve your aim, you'll experience enduring joy. Even Michael Phelps felt the letdown of reaching his goals and contemplated suicide after the 2012 Olympics, where he won four gold and two silver medals.[1]

Maybe you've lost weight and saw it wasn't everything you'd dreamed it would be. While it was fun to shop, you still found yourself enslaved to dietary adherence, fearful that the weight would come back and you'd be left still battling the same insecurities.

1. Christina Capatides, "Michael Phelps Opens Up About Depression, Says He Thought About Killing Himself After Olympics," *CBS News*, April 17, 2018, www.cbsnews.com/news/michael-phelps-reveals-he-suffered -from-depression-thought-about-killing-himself-after-olympics/.

Same here.

It wasn't until I found goals that motivated me on a deeper level, goals that anchored themselves in my values, that I could consistently make daily choices that were good for me. Healthy habits that come from a place of self-care and allegiance to what matters most to us far surpass those rooted in guilt, shame, and restriction, both in joy and sustainability.

To find real power behind your goals, you've got to have a *why* that motivates you in a profound and intrinsic way. This is done by connecting your goals to your values—the core of who you are and what matters most to you. Then you shape your goals around those values.

Getting Realistic with Your Goals

I used to loathe goal setting, and I still get a little squeamish hearing those words. I know; I'm a health coach, and I should believe that goals are the first step in any great transformation.

Ugh. There comes that feeling again. I just don't like feeling like a failure.

When setting goals, we tend to over- or undershoot. I used to be an overshooter. In my mind, I imagined that tomorrow would always be better. That I'd have more self-control, display greater discipline, and be able to walk through the bakery department without even making eye contact with a sweet. But, alas, my long-term goals were usually left in the wake of my short-term desires.

Those who tend to underestimate their abilities have the foresight to know how awful failure feels, and so they set the bar low or just cease to try at all. You may procrastinate or even label yourself as "lazy" because you just can't seem to get started. But you're not lazy; your goals are just letting you down.

My perception of goal-setting changed when I realized my lack of excitement was because I was chasing goals that (a) I actually didn't care about that much and (b) were completely out of my control. Intrigued? Yeah, I was too.

The Lord wired us for eternity while also admonishing us to focus on *this* day. It's a big-picture goal with a day-to-day application. As usual, it turns out any profitable perspective is rooted in God's Word.

Let's hone in on the reason you picked up this book. What do you want in your relationship with food and your body? Are you set on weight loss, or have you reached the point where food freedom is what you long for?

It's time to find out. This chapter will be a bit more interactive. But don't worry, it's not about getting it "right." It's about getting honest. When you take the time to quiet the noise and listen to yourself, you can learn much more about creating a sustainable, healthy lifestyle than you would studying and highlighting a shelf full of diet books. So grab a journal or open the notes app on your phone, and let's go.

Why Do You Want What You Want?

When it comes to health and fitness, what are your goals? You may want to lose a certain number of pounds, improve your blood work numbers, or be able to easily get up and down off the floor when playing with your kids or grandkids. These are all great and valid long-term goals—but let's go a bit deeper and look at your drive behind them. This will help you add a little fuel to the fire.

Jot down your initial thoughts regarding your goals. Don't overthink, just get them out of your head and onto paper so you can see them. Then I encourage you to steep on the two questions below, asking the Holy Spirit to give you the wisdom that only he can.

1. What are my health and fitness goals? What is the reason I want this?
2. What makes these changes so important to me? In what ways will they enhance my quality of life and happiness? What is the reason I want this?

As you dig beneath the surface, you may begin to find your more meaningful aspirations, the ones that reveal your real reasons for wanting to meet your goals. What you uncover may solidify your initial objective or make you see that you may need a more purposeful aim. For example, if your weight loss goals are all about gaining acceptance, you may realize that people are finicky and you actually care more about what God thinks about you. So you adjust your goal and decide it's more important to become rooted in your identity in Christ than it is to reach an elusive number on the scale. Of course, these kinds of shifts take time, patience, and a lot of prayer, so give yourself a ton of grace as you dive into your deeper goals—and always write them in pencil because you may change your mind again.

Move from Outcome Goals to Behavior Goals

Chances are that at least one of the goals you just wrote down—you know, the one you *really* want to accomplish—is beyond your control. Shocking, right? That's okay, we all do it. It's probably an outcome goal—your desired end result. Outcome goals are long-term objectives that target a specific result. They emphasize what you want to accomplish rather than the steps you'll take to get there.

Here's the reality: You can't simply *make* yourself lose weight, lower your A1C, or shave five minutes off your 5k. Even if you white-knuckle it and stay laser-focused, these outcomes are multifactorial and not directly within your realm of control.

Need proof? You've probably experienced this before: You did all the "right" things only to hop on the scale, get your blood work results, or cross the finish line painfully disappointed. What happened? You worked so hard. It's frustrating and disheartening. And this kind of shattered expectation can lead to some real self-sabotaging behavior.

The issue is we don't recognize what we can and can't control. Weight loss is nonlinear, genetics influence our blood markers, and sprained ankles happen. Today is the sum of our previous choices, and the gap between tomorrow and next year is paved with daily decisions.

When we try to control what's out of our control, we're in for an emotional roller coaster. But when we swap outcome goals for behavior goals, we finally have an aim that's within our grasp.

Outcome goals get us excited; behavior goals get us results.

If outcome goals state where we want to end up, behavior goals are the path to getting there. Let's say you want to increase your bone density. Hip fractures run in your family, and you'd like to be stronger before your fiftieth birthday. While increasing your bone density and gaining strength are fabulous goals, they happen in the future, in a time and space you cannot change today. Perhaps you get a bit more specific and measurable and decide you'd like to add half a point to your DEXA Scan score and be able to do ten push-ups without a break. While less elusive, those are still your end goals—outcome goals.

To find your *behavior* goals, consider what daily actions would likely take you where you want to go. You may decide you want to strength train three days a week for thirty minutes and perform two sets of push-ups on alternating days. Awesome! Now you've got a goal you can reach and be successful at, day in and day out.

When you choose doable habits, your confidence will grow, and you'll stay inspired on the road to your destination, especially if those aspirations support what you value most.

What Do You Value?

I'd just polished off the box of fudgesicles and felt terrible. Yes, I was stuffed and uncomfortable and regretting those last few bites I'd practically forced down. But, most of all, I felt awful on the inside. Of course there was the diet guilt, but this was something deeper, and I couldn't quite put my finger on it.

A few months later, a friend shared a personality quiz with me. Some of the questions inquired about my personal values, asking what qualities and characteristics I desired to reflect in my life. My top values have always been integrity, transparency, and reliability. Then it struck me—my unwanted eating habits were contradictory to what I valued. I was aiming for perfection (not a top value) and sacrificing my integrity by wavering between diet adherence and overeating. When I realized that eating with integrity could inspire me and my behavior goals, I was onto something powerful.

You are more than a body. In the last chapter, we discussed how God made you exactly as he desired. He designed your appearance—your curly hair, piercing eyes, or warm smile. He also wove a personality into your DNA—the way you're naturally sporty, good with numbers, or able to spot even the most subtle emotions in others. The Lord also gifted you hopes, dreams, and values to support your calling.

What you value determines how you spend your time, money, and talents. It's important to know what you hold dear so that you can filter your decision through that lens. When you act outside of your personal values, you'll probably feel pretty icky (and maybe even want to eat just to drown out the uncomfortable feelings). Embrace what matters to you so you can *do* what matters most.

When we talk about our personal values, we're referring to the principles, standards, and characteristics we hold dear. We feel the best when these values guide how we act, make decisions, *and* set goals. For example, if we value honesty and compassion, those traits will influence how we interact with others and what we strive for in life. It's like having a personal compass that helps us navigate our choices and behaviors.

However, we often forget to remember our values, especially when it comes to how we eat and how we look, as the voice of the world is noisier, flashier, and trendier than the still, small voice whispering in our hearts and minds. So, let's listen in!

What do *you* value? Review the list below and consider which are your top values. While you may find a dozen, stick to three if you can. Record them in your journal. You're looking for the best of the best— the qualities that ignite a fire in your heart and propel you to action.

If you have a hard time narrowing it down, visualize how each value would change how you spend your time. For example, if you cherish *service*, your weekends may be spent volunteering—but if *fun* is number one, you'll probably be playing board games with friends or your kids. Of course you can do both, but seeing how a value impacts your real life can help you to hone in on what's most important to you.

Core Values

Achievement	Discipline	Initiative	Respect
Adventure	Discretion	Integrity	Responsibility
Authenticity	Efficiency	Intimacy	Righteousness
Authority	Encouragement	Joy	Security
Autonomy	Enthusiasm	Justice	Self-control
Balance	Fairness	Kindness	Self-respect
Beauty	Faith	Knowledge	Service
Boldness	Fame	Leadership	Spirituality
Challenge	Flexibility	Learning	Stability
Charity	Friendships	Love	Status
Commitment	Fun	Loyalty	Success
Community	Generosity	Meaningfulness	Teachability
Compassion	Godliness	Meekness	Thoroughness
Competency	Goodness	Mercy	Thoughtfulness
Contentment	Grace	Openness	Trustworthiness
Contribution	Gratitude	Optimism	Wealth
Courage	Growth	Patience	Wisdom
Creativity	Happiness	Peace	Work
Curiosity	Honesty	Perseverance	
Dependability	Humility	Prudence	
Determination	Humor	Recognition	
Diligence	Influence	Reputation	

Got them written down? Great work! I know it's hard to narrow it down, but nothing is set in stone; we can change as people, and so can our top values. What you have is an excellent starting point.

Imagine what a life guided by these three values looks like. How would that change your relationships, how you spend your time, your goals . . . and your eating?

Merging Goals and Values

When I realized my top values were all about trustworthiness, it became clear to me that my goals needed a makeover. If my primary focus was to make myself look good on the outside, regardless of what was going on inside, then I was going to lack integrity. I needed an aim that supported my values—one that would inspire me to get back up, even after a rough day. I needed a goal that meant more to me than being shiny on the outside and shattered on the inside.

When you look at your goals, do they support your values? Do your goals and values feel compatible? It's important they are aligned; otherwise, you'll struggle to stay committed and wonder why. If it feels impossible to align the two, consider reevaluating your goals.

Embracing Your Values in Your Eating

So, how does this knowledge of goals and values impact your everyday life? How will knowing that you value generosity help you bypass your crunchy cravings after a stressful day with the kids?

Understanding your top values will help you recover from those less-than-ideal eating moments more easily. You'll see that you're no longer on a diet-tightwire but following a personally important track. You desire to operate with integrity, and that means getting back up because that's what feels virtuous to you.

Also, your daily habits can support your values by helping you feel your best. I think we all can agree that it's much easier to walk in joy, peace, and patience when we're well-fed and rested. When you start to weave your goals and values together, you ignite a victorious cycle!

Embracing Past Experiences in Your Eating

Now that you know what's important to you and where you want to go, it's time to look back at where you've been. I've done my share of diets, and I bet you have too. When I consider the lost time and money, I can't help but feel a sense of regret. I wish I'd seen the downward spiral before it accelerated to a blur, but I didn't . . . and maybe you didn't either. Praise God that he works even our dieting experiences for our good and his glory.

Take a moment to think about your diet history. There are likely plans you followed that make you giggle now (you know, like the one where you only ate eggs for a week) and some you'd like to forget about. But hidden among the sea of food lists and portion sizes are some treasures to be found. In fact, knowing what *doesn't* work is almost as important as knowing what *does*.

What plans have you been on? Review each one (or at least a handful of them) and determine what you liked and did not like about it. Some may have no positive points, and that's okay. But you may glean a few nuggets from others, such as realizing that you enjoyed eating less meat or found you couldn't live without it. Please be aware that there may be parts and pieces of certain programs that worked for you, while as a whole it was still all too much. For example, say a low-carb diet brought you weight loss and better energy, but it wasn't sustainable, and you missed bread far too much. Now you know that eating fewer carbs may be helpful, *and* it needs to be at a level you can live with.

Look deeper than the plan itself. Was it possible that something besides the actual eating regime was what led to your success or struggles? For example, maybe the best part of the program was that you ate at home more, cooked up your weekday lunches on Sundays, and had more veggies and lean protein in your diet. You can distill that planning a few homemade meals each week that include veggies and protein (and a carb too!) could be a really enjoyable practice for you. You may even double-up those recipes so your lunches are covered as well! Or maybe you enjoyed having a meal plan laid out for you but found the counting and calculating unbearable. You can glean that done-for-you meal plans could be a blessing but micromanaging is a burden.

Keep these concepts in mind as you move forward so that you can filter potential habits through this knowledge about what you like and what you don't. You are in the driver's seat.

Embracing Your Preferences in Your Eating

How do you desire to eat? If you could put *anything* on your plate, what would it be?

If you're scratching your head wondering why I'm asking you this, then you're in for a real treat.

If you've been around the dieting world for a while, you've seen how quickly trends can change and how oppositional they can be to one another. In the '90s we were avoiding fat and eating six small meals a day. Then the new millennium brought a fear of carbs. Following that trend, we found ourselves eating mostly fat and fewer meals, and then in the 2020s it became no meals at all for many hours at a time with intermittent fasting. Each new iteration has claimed to be "the best."

But is it really "the best" if it doesn't work for you?

The best is what is doable, sustainable, appealing, *and* effective. If you don't like eating the prescribed way, you won't do it for long. Maybe you gag when you eat cottage cheese or hate the texture of oatmeal. To base your week's breakfasts on either of these would be a really unkind thing to do to yourself. Especially when there are so many other delicious, healthy options out there.

It's time to embrace your preferences and see how validating your wants and needs can calm your eating anxieties. Consider the following questions. Do you prefer to . . .

Eat a smaller portion of richer food OR a larger portion of lighter food?

Eat less frequent, larger meals OR more frequent, smaller meals?

Eat all foods "in moderation" OR avoid particular foods that are challenging to navigate (for now)?

Imagine what would happen if you embraced your preferences and gave yourself permission to eat in a way that feels good physically, mentally, *and* emotionally to you.

"What feels good to *you*" is important to note, as we may assume what will feel good is what the flesh is asking for—but that's a crucial differentiation. My flesh may say that eating a gallon of ice cream would feel really good, but in reality I would be left overfull, unsatisfied, and disappointed.

On the flipside, we may assume that what we want should match up with what we think we *should* eat—the cumulative cross section of the foods our past diets have labeled as "good." In reality, trying to fit into such a narrow box would be anything but appealing and sustainable.

It's time to embrace *your* best way of eating—cue your Mind-Body Scan habit! As you may have noticed, your body is giving you feedback about how certain foods and portions work (or don't) for you. Consider how different meals make you feel, both physically and emotionally. How's your energy, focus, and satisfaction after eating?

Notice I said *meals* and not *foods*. While there are probably certain foods that make you feel great or not-so-great, avoid making blanket statements such as "Donuts make me feel bad, and salad makes me feel good." Nutrition is rarely that black-and-white. Notice the quantity and context. For example, ordering a small glazed donut alongside an egg frittata to enjoy with your family is miles apart from ordering three massive candy-coated donuts and sneak-eating them in the car before you get home.

Start to gather data about what you like and dislike, without judgment and without assumptions. Then, you'll use this information to inform your future eating paths and plans, creating a way to eat that works for you.

HABIT 4: SIMPLY PLAN AHEAD

Are you ready to see how you are going to start doing that now? It's time to learn your next habit: Simply Plan Ahead. You're one smart cookie, but when it comes to eating, you may be so used to following someone else's rules that you rarely pause to consider what actually works for *you*. You've tried to follow plans created by someone else, someone you've never met, but it feels stifling because it's not matched to your needs. Or maybe you got tired of micromanaging your food, so now you just eat on the fly, grabbing whatever is convenient.

It's time to shift gears and begin to create a way of eating that supports your goals, values, preferences, physical health, and spiritual growth. If that sounds like a lot, don't worry. You'll start out simple and, over time, choosing what to eat will become second nature.

Your habit this chapter is intended to give you the pause you deserve when deciding what to eat. However, there is zero expectation of perfection or proficiency. After all, our struggles are about more than just food. Even so, planning your meals will begin to even out unwanted food behaviors intensified by skipping meals, ignoring cravings, or forgetting to pack your lunch.

Simply Plan Ahead is a gentle habit that provides an opportunity to consider what you would *like* to eat, based on what you know about yourself so far. You'll take a few minutes in the morning (or the night before) to loosely plan what you'd like to eat for the day. No weighing or measuring, just a realistic intention to make sure you're well-fed. This practice is incredibly beneficial because you're never left scrounging the cabinets or "ordering" your lunch out of a vending machine.

When you plan ahead, you give yourself an opportunity to think clearly so your decisions are not rash or thoughtless. When our emotions are high, we're overly hungry, or we've already packed everybody else's lunch but ours, our decision-making abilities won't make the grade. But when we give ourselves the space and place to make a good decision, the chances are much higher that we will. The goal is simply *forethought*. When we think ahead, we're prepared to make better choices. Think of it as a gift to yourself.

If you're squirming, please don't. Simply Plan Ahead is meant to serve you, not the other way around. Just because you plan to eat something doesn't mean you always "have to" eat it. There's a learning curve, and flexibility is key.

Start by looking for a consistent three- to five-minute pocket of time to jot down your meals and snacks for the upcoming day. If you can anchor this action to another daily routine, you'll skyrocket your chances of success. For example, let's say you wind down in bed with a good book after you've done all your nighttime chores. To remind yourself to Simply Plan Ahead, you place a small journal that will hold your plans on top of your book. Or if you're a morning planner, perhaps you tuck your journal where you naturally start your day—whether that's by your Bible, your coffee maker, or your favorite window.

Now you're set to create a routine! Here's how to Simply Plan Ahead:

Step 1: Look ahead. What's on deck? Will you be home, at work, on the go, or a combo? What foods do you have available? Will you be eating with others? Do you need to pack or prep?

Step 2: Pick your plan. Based on the logistics of your day, what would you like to eat? What meals will adequately fuel you while also keeping you comfortable and ready to continue your day?

Step away from the knee-jerk reaction that comes from a place of dietary restriction ("Don't eat *that!*" or "Eat *all* that!") and think about what you'd enjoy eating and what would make you feel good.

I like to call this marrying your wants with wisdom. Don't feel too wise when it comes to eating? That's okay; you've proven you can make amazing decisions in other areas of your life, so now it's time to practice those skills in your eating. And let's not forget, if you've asked Jesus to be your Lord and Savior, the Holy Spirit—the Spirit of Truth (John 15:26), the Spirit of the living God (2 Cor. 3:3), the Helper (John 14:26)—resides within you. What a gift! You and

I can ask the Spirit for help in our everyday decisions, including what to eat.

So, how do you marry wants with wisdom? First, ask yourself what you would like to eat, then filter your response through the wisdom and guidance of the Holy Spirit. For example, let's say you ask yourself this question and the resounding answer is "Pizza, of course!" Now, what does your experience tell you about eating pizza? You've probably seen both extremes. You can picture yourself sitting around the table with your family, stabbing your chicken Caesar salad with irritation while they all enjoyed a cheesy slice. You may also remember times you ate too much—you had two slices while sitting at the table and felt guilty, and then sneakily ate another two slices when you were cleaning up. Not eating pizza is not fun, but neither is eating too much. To marry your wants with wisdom, you could decide to have one or two slices plus a side salad. This way, you'll enjoy the taste of your fave plus the lightness of some veggies. A total win-win!

If you're like me and could eat pizza every day, you may consider using that desire as a cue for meal planning, putting flatbread pizzas or another pizza-inspired dish on your lunch roster for the week. The same can go for tacos, waffles, or any food that you enjoy eating but know it's not a dish to eat every day. Give it a healthy makeover when you put it on repeat and then *have* the real deal, with wisdom.

As you continue to read and implement what you learn in this book, you'll have more and more tools to apply to your daily eating, so please don't become discouraged if some days your plans just don't stick. The key when you Simply Plan Ahead is to uncover what factors come into play on those hard days.

You may be facing a practical, emotional, or spiritual challenge. Let's look at some of those now.

Planning Challenge #1: Your Plans Change

Life happens, and God is on the move. Some days just simply don't go as planned. It's important to be flexible enough to go with the flow so that changes don't make you feel out of control. No matter where you are, you can pray for the wisdom to make a choice that feels great. If you get a flat tire and are stuck at a rural gas station well past lunchtime, your best option may be a smaller portion of greasy food or a bag of sugarcoated trail mix.

It's okay. Eat it and move on.

Learn what you can, and you'll begin to have go-to swaps for those less-than-ideal days.

Planning Challenge #2: You Don't Want to Eat What You Planned

Last night you thought you wanted those delicious dinner leftovers for lunch, but now you're in the mood for something else. You can navigate this in one of two ways. Both are excellent, so pray and be led by your peace.

1. Change your plans and marry your wants with wisdom. This is a great option if you've been denying yourself what you like to eat (even if only in your mind) for a long time. It's validating to truly listen and to meet your desires and needs with wisdom.

2. Plan it for tomorrow. Take note of the new, tasty idea you had and add it to an upcoming menu. This is a great option if you've felt bossed around by your flesh or if you have a propensity to see and eat without thinking. When you save it for tomorrow, you're validating your wants but not being reactive. With a planned pause, you'll have some time to decide what you'd really like while also growing your self-control.

Planning Challenge #3: You're Feeling Emotional

If you've used food to cope with stress, it's unrealistic to expect yourself to suddenly stop just because you made a plan. Growing out of emotional eating takes time and new skills. We'll talk about how to navigate those emotions in a later chapter. In the meantime, if you have a moment when the need to soothe yourself through your eating eclipses all else, then do the next best thing and learn what you can about your triggers. Food is not the problem, so find out what is.

When you decide to emotionally eat, grab a notebook first. What you're feeling in that moment of weakness is a gold mine of valuable data about what pushes you to eat. Jot down what you've been thinking about that day. What thoughts have been playing like a broken record, weighing heavily on your heart and mind? Can you identify any feelings, fears, or anxieties? Take note, eat, and move on. Beating yourself up will only keep you stuck in a vicious cycle. Give yourself *grace*—you and the Lord are going to get to the root and pluck it out!

We have a real, prowling enemy looking to steal our joy by any means possible. If you feel the fiery dart coming your way, take up the shield of faith (Eph. 6:16) by going to God's Word and finding promises that speak to your situation. Search the Scriptures for a word that resounds in your heart and speak it out. God's Word will change the environment, inside of us and around us!

PERSONALIZE YOUR HABIT

Are you ready to pick your starting point? As described above, Simply Plan Ahead is about planning each day's meals and snacks. However, choosing a habit that is doable, sustainable, appealing, and effective is key. If you can't do it, can't do it for as long as you need to, or don't want to do it, it's time to change it up!

This is where you exercise your autonomy and find a habit that fits you and your lifestyle. Not what you *think* will work, not what you *wish* would work, but a habit you can nail, just about every day. You may adjust Simply Plan Ahead by going micro, starting with one meal a day and then building from there. Or you might go macro by doing some general meal planning for yourself and your family.

Let's say that the afternoon is your kryptonite. You may benefit most by planning your lunch and afternoon snack, aiming to make both tasty and satisfying. Or maybe you don't have a meal plan at all, and you realize that picking up what you need at the store for nourishing breakfasts and a few dinners a week would be incredibly helpful for you. Start there!

You'll practice this habit for the next week (or longer, if you want to take time to really let it sink in). Be sure to use your habit tracker and follow along with the included Scripture writing journal to keep your new habit and Jesus-first focus front and center.

Uncovering Your Design

"What do *you* like to do?"

I dreaded this question at social gatherings. *Can we please talk about the weather or your dog? I'd love to hear about your dog,* I'd think as I tried to guide the conversation in a different direction. Why was I so resistant to this seemingly harmless question? I mean, isn't asking about hobbies a great way to get to know one another?

The truth is, I didn't know what I liked to do. I had no hobbies. I spent my free time exercising, managing what I ate, and overeating. I'd always felt like a bit of an oddball. When I was a teen, my friends would head out at 8:00 p.m. to catch a movie, and I'd pass on their invitations to join so I could go to bed at 9:00. I prefer solitude over parties and organizing my closet over a trip to the beach.

Weird, right? Who likes Staples better than the spa? Me. And I'm cool with it . . . now.

God intends to use every part of our personalities and preferences to further his kingdom. When he made you, he created you with a purpose. In order for you to fulfill that purpose, you're going to need some gifts and strengths to get there. But guess what? Every single gift and every single strength has its weaknesses. Yep—part of your design includes things you don't like or that you're not good at.

> If God has given you the gift of empathy, you can find the one person in a crowd who needs encouragement, but your sensitivity may also mean your feelings get hurt when a stranger cuts you off in traffic.
>
> If you're decisive and focused, you're an awesome leader, but you may err on the side of bossy if you're not careful.
>
> If your friends know you as the fun one who brings laughter, joy, and spontaneity to the group, they probably know your tardiness is also part of the package.

While this chapter has honed in on your eating preferences, let your new acknowledgments here begin to translate into other areas of your life, too, as you aspire to know how you're wired, so that you can live with passion and purpose. Imagine how your life would change if you allowed yourself to be authentically *you*. The taste of fulfillment would diminish the draw of lesser things.

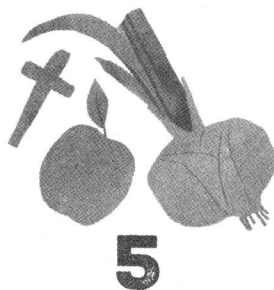

GROW FRUITFUL HABITS

*But the fruit of the Spirit is love, joy, peace, patience,
kindness, goodness, faithfulness, gentleness, self-control;
against such things there is no law.*

Galatians 5:22–23

My hands were stained, my legs looked tie-dyed, and my towels
were ruined.

I thought it was a good idea; the label and the advertisements
both said it was easy to apply. The process sounded foolproof—just
a few swipes of this magic cream, and I'd wake up looking like I'd
spent the week on the beaches of Hawaii. But now I was covering
up my splotchy legs due to my self-tanner fail.

I tossed the bottle in the trash without a second thought, irritated with the product's performance. I didn't take the failure
personally, and I didn't wring my hands over my lack of self-tanner
application skills. I simply saw that it didn't work out as I had
planned and moved on, albeit temporarily a little more orange
than before.

That's the nature of new ventures. While we try to choose the best route possible, we often don't know the outcome the endeavor will produce until we try it. In this case, the only "fruit" the self-tanner produced in my life was a lovely mottled shade of orange.

Despite my self-tanner episode, I've always been a pretty decent decision-maker, especially when it comes to stopping something that clearly doesn't work. You probably are too! If you go to a doctor and she only makes your symptoms worse, you change docs as fast as your little fingers can dial the phone. If your mechanic finds more problems than parts, you're on the hunt for a new car before you can say "lemon." No wavering, no wondering, just clear decisions.

But when it comes to dieting, we're blinded by the inflated promises that coax us into thinking the next one is the answer we've been waiting for. We kept going, trying to fix the problem with the very thing that induced it, hoping for a different result—the definition of insanity.

I started my first diet hoping for greater self-confidence, but my dieting career only produced an obsession with food, infertility, a trip to the emergency room due to diet pills, a six-week visit to an eating disorder treatment center (over Christmas), and countless therapy sessions. Definitely not what I'd signed up for. But because I thought I was the weak link, I kept going.

Oh, how I wish I'd noticed the correlation and taken an impartial look at the outcome. Maybe then I would've changed course sooner, putting my attention and effort into something *fruitful*.

The Standard for Fruitfulness

Nobody likes a bad investment. We want to put our time, energy, and resources into profitable endeavors that produce a gain, whether it's increased health, happiness, or hope. Even tough times can bring about beneficial results if we allow the Lord to use them to prune us, to make us more like Jesus. In the same way, our daily activities, routines, and even mundane tasks can be used for our good and his glory, bearing fruit.

But we often don't hold the inputs and influences in our lives to a high enough standard of fruitfulness.

When we talk about fruit, we're talking about the results our actions produce. Think about the fruit of brushing your teeth, walking the dog, or zoning out on social media. Do those habits produce sweet, sour, bland, or rotten fruit?

It's important to note that because our habits and routines impact our overall well-being—spirit, soul, and body—fruitful habits equal fruitful humans. In the Bible, the production of fruit indicates the health of a tree or an individual because fruit is the product of nourishment. In trees, it's good soil, sufficient water, and adequate sunshine. In human beings, it's being rooted in God's Word, refreshed by the Holy Spirit, and warmed by God's unconditional love and grace.

It's worth noting that fruit is not for the trees' consumption. While fruit is a byproduct of good care and favorable conditions, those apples and oranges hanging from their branches are for others to benefit from.

Did you catch that?

The Lord wants you to be so full, nourished, and *well* that you have excess for others to feed on. Imagine what would happen if you held your dietary habits, exercise routines, and pastimes to a standard of fruitfulness. Not self-effort-soaked production. Not white-knuckling. But seeking-God-first fruitfulness.

Because when you were created as a child of God, you were made to bear fruit.

You Were Made to Be Fruitful

I've always had a bent toward negativity; I was born a glass-half-empty kind of gal, especially in how I saw myself. When I looked at myself, all I could see were mishaps and mistakes, from my appearance to my performance. I believed that the only way I could be good enough was to be the best at any and every pursuit. So I tried my hardest to be number one and nothing less. Or . . . I'd quit. It was all about me and what I could do. How I looked and what others thought about me. Me, me, me.

And because we're human, anytime we look solely at ourselves, we're bound to find shortcomings and mistakes. But this isn't news to God. He knew before the foundation of the world that we would never measure up to his perfect standard of holiness. Yet, in his infinite love and mercy, he made a way. God sent his Son not to scold or shame us but to rescue us. Jesus came to live among us, to understand our struggles, and to offer us grace upon grace.

Through the life, death, and resurrection of Jesus, God bridged the gap we could never cross on our own. And now, instead of striving for perfection, we get to walk in relationship with the One who is perfect and who welcomes us, flaws and all, into his presence with open arms.

So, why are we so shocked when we miss the mark?

It's the enemy who whispers in our ears, telling us that we're not good enough or that we've made too many mistakes to be used by God. But those are just lies intended to keep us stuck and focused on ourselves and not our awesome and wonderful God, who created us to bear fruit in every good work (Col. 1:10). In *every* area of our lives.

For too long, we've allowed ourselves to engage in fruitless ventures, especially in our dieting. These pursuits have taken more than they've given, drained our energy, and been used by the devil to steal our joy. And it's gone on long enough.

As a daughter of the King, you can have a royal standard, expecting your ventures and pursuits to meet a high level of fruitfulness when they're yielded to the guidance, direction, and occasional pruning from our loving heavenly Father. It's time to get picky about your habits and begin to discern whether a "healthy habit" is actually good for *you* based on its fruit—the results it produces in your life. No wavering, no wondering, just clear decisions. When fruitfulness becomes the gatekeeper of your endeavors, you'll experience a newfound clarity and confidence in distinguishing what works and what doesn't.

How to Spot Fruitful Habits

So, how do we know if our habits are making the grade? How do we assess if our daily behaviors are beneficial? We start by noticing the fruit they produce! A fruitful habit is one that helps to support the development of the fruit of the Spirit in our lives. Galatians 5:22–23 states: "But the fruit of the Spirit is love, joy, peace, patience, kindness, goodness, faithfulness, gentleness, self-control; against such things there is no law."

While the fruit is a gift, our behaviors can create a nurturing *or* stifling environment. While the connection won't always be linear or obvious, we're looking for an underlying trend of growth. You probably won't say, "I ate broccoli and now I'm more joyful," but you may notice that eating more produce, with all its nutritional benefits, helps you feel more satisfied and less snacky after meals. Over time, these seemingly small shifts can lighten your load and lift your spirit—because when your habits support your well-being, joy starts to take root.

Let's take a look at your dieting history again. What was the fruit produced in your life by restrictive diets? Can you recognize the fruit of the Spirit? I can tell you that micromanaging my eating left me feeling anything but fruitful.

In contrast, how does it feel when you practice your Grow in Gratitude or Sowing Seeds of Self-Control habit? When habits are done for God's glory and by God's strength, they produce a noticeably different outcome. Let's see if you can spot the fruit of the Spirit or the works of the flesh (Gal. 5:19–23) in the table below.

Dieting vs. Food Freedom

Fruit of the Spirit	Restrictive Diets	Food Freedom
Love	When following diets, my primary concern is what I can eat and what I am going to eat. I take the best pieces, prioritize my meals, and even get upset when others eat my allotted food.	When my primary concern is adopting a healthy habit for my good and God's glory, I talk to him more and feel more aligned with his will.
Joy		Unencumbered, I find myself praying for others and being more aware of God's leading in my daily life.
Peace	I am irritable and frustrated when I don't follow my food plan correctly and more prone to snap at my loved ones.	Interacting with the Lord helps me feel more loving, joyful, peaceful, patient, and kind.
Patience	When the scale doesn't cooperate, I get angry. All of this leaves me steeped in guilt and shame, feeling embarrassed by my behavior.	When I eat with God in mind, I trust that he will provide for me because he loves me. I can pray about what to eat and be led by my peace.
Kindness		
Goodness	Each diet leaves me a little less faithful, unable to stay committed to what I've started.	When I am fueling myself well, choosing foods that I enjoy (God made ice cream too!) while also making wise choices, I'm more even-keeled physically, mentally, and emotionally.
Faithfulness	While I may look like the "healthy" girl to watching eyes, in secret my eating is out of control. I run to food for everything—partly because I fear it will be taken away and partly because it is my comfort. The dishonesty leaves me in turmoil and despair.	If I slip and eat in a way that I'd not planned, I run to God and ask him to help me make a better choice next time. His unconditional love and grace fill my heart with praise! It feels amazing to partner with the Lord and allow him to develop the spirit of self-control within me!
Gentleness		
Self-Control		

Yowza! Did you catch that? Can you see the polarizing difference between self-focused diets and Spirit-led eating? While it takes time and patience to shift gears, the journey alone will bring you closer to the Lord as you develop habits that improve your health and move you toward your long-term goals.

If stepping away from diets makes you feel nervous, I understand. That's normal. The unknown can be scary, so let's focus on what you do know: God is good, he wants what's best for you, and your diet-management skills aren't getting you where you want to go. If you're starting to catch the vision of Fruitful Habits, I bet you're wondering how to get started. Let's look at the practical side of this spiritually rooted practice. It's a big-picture goal with a day-to-day application.

Sustainable Farming

You and I are good at starting diets. We have the bookshelves and bank debits to prove it. Yet if our eating goals aren't easy to incorporate into our daily routine, we won't keep up with them and they won't be successful. Real change hinges on consistency—and consistency is only possible with sustainability. That's how habits are made.

But even the best-laid plans won't cause us to be fruitful without Christ.

This reminds me of John 15:4–5:

Abide in me, and I in you. As the branch cannot bear fruit by itself, unless it abides in the vine, neither can you, unless you abide in me. I am the vine; you are the branches. Whoever abides in me and I in him, he it is that bears much fruit, for apart from me you can do nothing.

It all comes back to being rooted in God, a daily connection that inspires and empowers you to keep going, even and especially on hard days. Power from the Lord paired with practical knowledge is what will make your habits stick.

In the last chapter, we discussed how important it is to choose habits that are doable, sustainable, appealing, and effective. With that in mind, let's look at how sustainability can be supported with three practical and helpful assessments. When you review these sections, you'll see why your dietary change ventures may not have worked for you in the past.

But first, I want to encourage you to look at the points below as gentle guidance, *not* a set of unyielding rules. These resources are intended to help you, not complicate your life with extra to-dos. Remember, God is the Lord of your transformation. Do what you can and trust that he will meet you where you are, guiding you in creating sustainable, fruitful habits.

That's grace.

Develop Rooted Habits

Sustainable habits are the ones that find a home in our routines. Trees extend their roots deep into the soil for nourishment, but these roots also provide stability, anchoring the trees firmly and protecting them from toppling over during storms. To create rooted habits, we're looking to piggyback our new habits onto existing ones.

You've already started doing this through the previous chapters, but now it's time to get even more intentional. When adding a new habit, consider your current habits and routines. What do you do most days? Those are the patterns you want to look for.

Now, you may feel like your schedule is unpredictable and inconsistent, but there are always things you do most days. For example, regardless of the exact time, more often than not you make your bed, take a shower, brush your teeth, make coffee, read your Bible, eat breakfast, walk the dog, drive to work, eat lunch, visit the bathroom, pick up the kids, start a load of laundry, feed the dog, make dinner, and wash your face. These consistencies are all helpful anchors for new habits. If you tie in a new habit to one that already exists, you'll skyrocket your chances of success!

Count the Cost

Sustainable habits are the ones we find worth the investment of our time, energy, and effort. When going on a new diet or starting a new exercise routine, we tend to jump right in, assuming the new plan or program will fit right into our lifestyle. But our lives and routines have deep grooves worn from repetition, and we can't switch lanes on a moment's notice. With any new venture, there'll be adjustments to be made, and we'll need an honest assessment to determine whether we can or even want to make those changes. Scripture calls this counting the cost. "For which of you, desiring to build a tower, does not first sit down and count the cost, whether he has enough to complete it?" (Luke 14:28).

Our habits, helpful and unhelpful alike, will cost us something. Not every healthy change will come with a heavy set of costs, but each will likely cost something: comfort, ease, convenience, and so on. And that's not a negative thing—we make trades every day. But we rarely take the time to assess whether the cost paid is worth the value received.

Prepare for Challenges

Sustainable habits are flexible habits that stretch and adapt. When it came to my eating, I always believed that tomorrow would be easier. The self-control fairy would come, and I'd float through the day, nailing my diet despite any resistance. While that may sound like positive thinking, it was a daydream that set me up for heartache and disappointment.

Life happens, and our best plans get tossed by the wayside. If we're too attached to those plans, our habits won't fit into our day's reality. When choosing habits, it's important to have a backup plan. By considering potential opposition, you won't be surprised by bumps along the way. In fact, giving them some forethought helps your brain be better prepared to go into a solution-oriented mode, knowing that there's always a next best option and after that another, and another.

Even if only a trace of your original habit exists in your day, you've still prioritized its practice and created a placeholder to make tomorrow easier.

HABIT 5: GROW FRUITFUL HABITS

Time is precious, and energy is finite. We don't have the time or energy to waste on fruitless ventures. Now is the time to set a higher standard for habits, choosing only those we deem valuable, worth our effort, and fruitful. Habits that support us in our callings, whether within our neighborhood or across the ocean.

What are Fruitful Habits? As you've seen, Fruitful Habits are those that help to cultivate the gift of the fruit of the Spirit in your life. These are daily routines and practices that benefit you physically, mentally, and spiritually. Because you're choosing small, sustainable habits—seeds—it will take time to see the harvest of your efforts. But you'll know if what you're doing is working for you (or not) based on your fruit.

The best habits are those that have a positive ripple effect in your life. They help you get to the root of a struggle and not get hung up on unnecessary details that bog you down and sap your energy. You can stop overthinking tiny details that add stress to your eating, like whether to get whole grain or whole wheat bread. Instead, focus on the deeper need, such as allowing yourself to take a twenty-minute power nap in the afternoon when you tend to start grazing the kitchen, looking for a sugar rush.

Imagine the fruit you could cultivate by praying every time you enter the kitchen. While it is not a food-focused habit, you'll be talking to the Lord more when you need to the most. Or how about the fruit of going to bed thirty minutes earlier, adding more veggies to your dinner, or drinking more water? The possibilities are endless, as the only criteria for a Fruitful Habit is that you value what it produces.

Before you pick your habit, consider a few examples. Again, this is not a to-do list but is designed to inspire you. You'll find several ideas to pull from, but really, the sky's the limit. I'll also share some potential outcomes so you can envision how the habit may or may not work for you. Ultimately, I encourage you to follow the prompting of the Holy Spirit within you and be led by your peace.

- **Pray before meals.** Besides the awesome benefits of prayer, the pause before a meal offers you a moment to slow down, check in, and even do a Mind-Body Scan.
- **Drink more water.** Increasing your water intake, if needed, can help to reduce cravings and boost your energy levels by keeping your body hydrated and functioning optimally.
- **Eat more veggies.** Low in calories and high in fiber, vitamins, and minerals, veggies will help you feel fuller at meals, crowding out less healthy eats.
- **Walk after dinner.** Movement after a meal will help to regulate your blood sugar while also getting you out of the kitchen as your food settles, leaving you fully satisfied.
- **Eat a balanced, whole-food breakfast.** Starting the day with real food will help avert unnecessary cravings and give you the focus you need to get things done!
- **Unplug on purpose.** If you tend to turn to food when you're physically tired or mentally exhausted, or to "treat" yourself, proactively planning a time to relax, pursue a hobby, or get to bed early (or on time) could help you meet your need to rest before you start to eat to occupy yourself.
- **Take a time-out.** If you struggle with emotional eating, it's important to understand the thoughts, feelings, and emotions that drive you to food. Prior to eating outside of your routine meals, commit to pausing for three minutes to pay attention, pray, and take note of what's happening in your heart and mind. This time-out will help you gather data so you can address your root issue rather than always trying to fix your eating.

Do you notice how each of these habits, while simple, could have a ripple effect into other areas of your life? When we broaden our vision and think more about the fruit of a habit than the tiny details, we stop adding food stress and set the stage for positive routines that can stick around for a lifetime.

PERSONALIZE YOUR HABIT

Now it's your turn. Did any of those habit ideas sound doable, appealing, and effective to you? Did they spur on a different idea? If you're already excited about an option, start there.

If you're not too sure, take a moment to consider your everyday life. Is there a particular time of day that's a struggle for you? Is there one routine or habit that's causing you a lot of angst? If so, zoom out and view your day as a big picture. How could you take better care of yourself so that you're better equipped to navigate that particular challenge when it comes up?

If you're still not sure, start with a habit on the list that feels doable, appealing, and effective. Then test it out, see how it fits, and adjust as needed. Be sure to choose a specific practice, such as walking after dinner on Monday, Wednesday, and Friday, or unplugging for fifteen minutes after you get home from work before diving into your afternoon routine. Having clarity on what you're doing will make it easier to plan for your progress.

Before we move on, let's take a moment to assess the skills learned above and make sure your habit is sustainable.

1. Is your Fruitful Habit rooted? How can you use an existing habit or routine to anchor your new habit?

   If your aim is to drink more water, you may want to fill up your bottle each time you prepare a meal. To remind yourself, consider placing a sticky note on the fridge near the water dispenser if you have one.

2. Have you counted the cost? Is this habit worth it to you? Let's say you decided you'd like to stop drinking soda but then realized you'll really miss it on pizza night. You may modify your habit to allow for two sodas a week and then find a soda alternative, such as herbal iced tea, when you're craving some flavor at other times.

3. Are you prepared? If life gets in the way of your habit, what's the backup plan? If you'd like to eat more vegetables but realize sometimes you run out of time to prep, try adding a few dollars to your grocery budget for precut produce—and grab some frozen options too.

After reviewing these three questions, on a scale of 1–10, what's your habit confidence? If you're at less than an 8, adjust your habit to make it easier. You may reduce the frequency, lessen the intensity by choosing fewer days or less time, or add in greater flexibility.

Do you see what you did? You self-coached yourself like some of the best coaches in the world, considering how to set yourself up for success.

Now you need one final thing: grace.

Remember, it is that unhelpful diet mindset that expects you to complete a plan perfectly. Habits are things done *most* of the time. If you find out your habit is too hard, you can change it. If life happens, you can encourage yourself to try again. Grace will only make your habit adoption more likely.

Okay, got your habit? You'll practice it for the next week (or longer, if you want to take time to really let it sink in). Be sure to use your habit tracker and follow along with the included Scripture writing pages to keep your habit and Jesus-first focus front and center.

Fruitful Living

I walked in the front door and made a beeline to the fridge, just like I had so many times before. I suspect the flooring was worn from my unwanted but obligatory routine. I was home—exhausted and picked clean, with nothing left to give. Not a thread of physical, emotional, or mental energy was left after my long (but pretty average) day.

My body wasn't asking for food, but I needed something—anything—to fill me up. So I ate. But because my lack was not nutritional, my hunger never subsided, and I just kept on eating. No peace, no joy . . . no fruit. And surely, no abundance to share.

But none of that was by accident. It's the enemy's plan to steal our joy because our freedom is about so much more than you or me. If he can keep us self-centered and self-condemning, we'll be too horizontally focused to bear the fruit of the Spirit. When we are disconnected from the vine, the worries of the world will choke God's Word in our hearts and minds (Mark 4:18–19).

But when we are connected to the vine, allowing the peace of Christ to guard our hearts and minds (Col. 3:15), we'll have fruit enough to share so that others can taste and see that the Lord is good (Ps. 34:8). In a dying and hurting world, joy and peace are the hottest commodities.

With this in mind, continue to focus your gaze on Jesus, seeking him for the strength and mercy you need to walk the path to food freedom. Then, as others see your fruitfulness and follow your gaze, you'll be pointing them to the only One who can meet their deepest needs too.

6

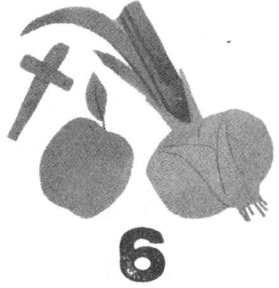

LET GO OF WHAT
HOLDS YOU BACK

*We destroy arguments and every lofty opinion raised
against the knowledge of God, and take every thought
captive to obey Christ.*

2 Corinthians 10:5

My heart raced with panic then sank with dread when I remembered what I had forgotten to do, opening a floodgate of negative self-talk.

You can't do anything right.

You should've known better.

Everyone is going to be disappointed in you.

On and on it went. By the time I walked through my front door at the end of the day, I was beaten and bruised, desperate for a reprieve from myself. *I need a treat*, I concluded. Just the mere thought brought a sigh of relief. I grabbed a spoon, opened the freezer, and pulled out the tub of Fudge Royal ice cream. The first mouthful was dreamy, the second pretty good, and then the negative self-talk resurfaced, reminding me that I'd promised my-self I was going to eat better today.

Ugh, I'm addicted to sugar. I have to do something about this.

So I swore off sugar for the thirty-seventh time.

It wasn't just about sugar. When sugar became off-limits, I would just find another vice: bread, cereal, pretzels, all kinds of carbs. So then I'd cut out carbs and find myself overdoing yogurt, protein powder, and fruit—eating bizarre mixtures of "zero-point" or low-calorie foods until the thought of another bite was nauseating.

I was overwhelmed by my lack of self-control and didn't know what else to do. But what confused me the most was that I had sig-nificant self-control in other areas of my life. I paid my bills on time, held a job, and cleaned the bathroom when I'd rather watch TV.

What was different about food?

The difference was the story I was telling myself. I believed food could soothe my wounds, and I was convinced that I had no discipline in my eating. So I lived like it.

My beliefs painted the reality I resided in, and I was caught in a gridlock of limiting beliefs and self-sabotaging thoughts. But what if I could change the narrative and start telling myself the truth—the truth God says about me—and act on it?

What if I wrote a new story?

The Stories We Tell

Whether you realize it or not, you are a master storyteller.

In fact, you've probably told yourself stories so epic, so thrilling, so filled with betrayal and deception they could rival any box office hit. Ah, the power of our minds. What a blessing our inquisitive nature and imagination can be—until they're used by the enemy to utterly exhaust us. Our histories give us plenty of content to create an unexpected plot twist, having had our share of heartbreak and adversity. And without God's Word to serve as a plumb line to these pictures, what we're viewing is an anxiety-inducing assumption.

Because the thinking part of our brain is quite computer-like, it takes the data we deliver through our thoughts and the emotions those thoughts evoke to shape our perception of reality. That's why two people can go through very similar circumstances and have vastly different outcomes—one thriving despite opposition and the other surrendering to it.

Your food struggles live in a story. Your past has influenced your beliefs about your relationship with food. However, that past is soaked with deceptions designed by Satan to keep you stuck in his virtual reality, one where you're at the mercy of your cravings, stranded, trying to manage this food thing on your own. One lacking the power of the Holy Spirit—the One who raised Christ from the dead—working in your life.

Those stories create two side effects we're going to address in this chapter, two ways of thinking that, when aligned with God's Word, will pave the way for you to walk out of this mess and into the food freedom Christ bought for you. We're going to talk about limiting beliefs and sabotaging thoughts—what they are, how they trip you up, and how you can rewrite them in a way that inspires and empowers you.

Limiting Beliefs

Limiting beliefs are those ideas we cling to that hold us back. They're like invisible rules we think we have to follow. These are beliefs about our abilities, what we deserve, or what's possible for us.

These beliefs usually come from your past experiences or messages you've picked up from the world around you. Like sticky weed seeds that hitchhike on your socks, you often don't know they're there until they hinder you. For instance, you might think you're not smart enough for your dream job, or that true joy is for everyone else but you. These kinds of thoughts can stop you from trying new things or stepping out in faith to claim the food freedom Christ's blood purchased for you.

And it's not like you want to stay stuck, but familiarity is comfortable. Your limiting beliefs, while tight like your eighth-grade jeans, are normal. Stepping out of your comfort zone can feel uncertain and scary. That's why when you try to move forward, something snaps you back like a rubber band pulled beyond its stretchiness—that's your limiting beliefs.

But how is *that* comfortable? Well, adopting and owning a label that lowers our standards can be a form of self-protection. Much like the way we may quit some things before we even start. It just seems easier and less painful not to try than to strive and fail.

If you believe you'll *never* be free of your struggle with sugar, then you'll be less heartbroken when you swear off sweets but cave and eat them anyway.

If you believe you'll *always* struggle with your weight, then you'll *never* have to push yourself harder than you feel comfortable—or you can *always* feel protected.

Can you see how limiting beliefs love absolutes like *can't, always, never, only,* and *must*?

When you say "I can't" or "I never," it tends to shut down possibilities and reinforces the idea that something is beyond your capability or completely unachievable.

Limiting beliefs aren't confined to "big" things; they show up everywhere. You may tell yourself that you loathe vegetables, despise exercise, don't like to cook, or can't go to the gym until you lose weight. Even these seemingly insignificant beliefs can keep you from doing the very things that will help you break through the bigger ones.

But there's more to the story than food. Limiting beliefs about your relationships, your career, your value, or whatever can show up in your eating as you look for comfort in a bowl of creamy mac and cheese or unleash your frustrations on a bag of crunchy chips.

It's all a grand scheme by the enemy, who wants to keep you shackled with imaginary chains of disbelief, thinking you are defined by your past. But if your previous or present experiences don't line up with what God says, then it's time to ditch those deceptions and think higher (Isa. 55:8–9). You were crafted with thoughtfulness (Ps. 139:13–14), created with a purpose (Eph. 2:10), and set free by Christ so you can live a life of freedom (Gal. 5:1). It's time to release those beliefs that contradict what the Lord says and to make your brain a blessing by renewing your mind.

Sabotaging Thoughts

Why do we sabotage ourselves when life is already tough enough without our interference? To sabotage something is to purposefully destroy, damage, or obstruct it, especially for political or military advantage.

The battle for our hearts begins in our minds.

Sabotaging thoughts are those that convince you to make choices to feed your flesh rather than your spirit. They are so tiny and feel so inconsequential in the moment that it's easy to let them slide in.

Our limiting beliefs are telling us a story, and our sabotaging thoughts act as justifications or rationalizations that help maintain those limiting beliefs by prodding actions that align with them, effectively ensuring the narrative continues as expected. For instance, a sabotaging thought like *I'll just have one* can justify giving in to a temptation, thereby reinforcing a limiting belief about how we lack self-control.

Sabotaging thoughts can also emerge as a way to excuse eating as a means of soothing our unmet needs or unruly emotions. Discomfort comes, and we'll find any reason to eat to temporarily calm the chaos—a seemingly innocent gateway that frequently begins with the phrase "I'll just."

I'll just eat the crumbs.

I'll just have one.

I'll just start tomorrow.

101

We crack the door open, and the story plays on as it has many times before. Like a savvy marketer peddling the latest pharmaceutical, we've told ourselves only the dreamy outcome and neglected to examine the fine print documenting the nightmarish side effects. "Just the crumbs" becomes the whole cake, "just one" turns into "just one more" until the box is gone, and tomorrow never comes. When we don't think beyond the temporary relief of the moment, we take the bait—hook, line, and sinker.

And while it's painful to notice your justifications, please don't let condemnation slip in. This is noble work you're doing here. We all get stuck in sabotaging thoughts, but only those who notice them can change them. And this one small, strategic exchange is life-altering.

Imagine what it would be like to catch a sabotaging thought, scrutinize it, and renew it before the desire gives birth to the very thing you're trying to avoid (James 1:14–15). It's time to think higher, rewrite those unhelpful thoughts, and make your mind an ally.

HABIT 6: FRUIT-FILLED JOURNALING

We're busy people, and much of our lives can be spent on autopilot. We get up, go to the bathroom, brush our teeth, make our coffee, and scroll social media, all with little conscious thought. You know what else we tend not to think about? Our thoughts! Yep, those beautiful little brains of ours are like unsupervised toddlers with crayons, sketching whatever they want, wherever they want.

The Bible makes it crystal clear that our thoughts are worth thinking about. We're even told to war with any thought that contradicts the knowledge of God because we are in a spiritual battle (2 Cor. 10:5).

Your habit this chapter is Fruit-Filled Journaling, a conscious practice where you'll strategically examine the beliefs and thoughts that are holding you back and hold them to biblical standards.

Much like the Mind-Body Scan (notice, name, and note), with Fruit-Filled Journaling you're going to notice your limiting beliefs and sabotaging thoughts, name them as fruitful or not, and renew them with alternative thoughts if needed.

This simple but powerful process provides the time and space you need to reprogram those unhelpful whims or ruminations with lifegiving, Holy Spirit–inspired scriptural convictions. Essentially, Fruit-Filled Journaling is Romans 12:2 in action: "Do not be conformed to this world, but be transformed by the renewal of your mind, that by testing you may discern what is the will of God, what is good and acceptable and perfect."

Step 1: Notice

Your first step is to write it down. Get any thought you want to examine out of your head and onto paper (or your notes app). Aside from helping you with your habit, writing will relieve some of the mental chaos, allow you to pray over your list, and help you discover your common thinking patterns.

To get the most benefit from this habit, notice all types of thoughts, not just the ones about food and your body. Beliefs or thoughts about your worth, value, performance, to-do list, expectations, relationships, or responsibilities can lead to an unrestful mental state that may result in seeking solace in food.

Not sure what you're thinking and feeling? No problem— noticing is a skill. You'll get there with practice. In the meantime, here are a few questions you can ask yourself:

Do I notice any limiting beliefs or sabotaging thoughts?
(Review the lists in the appendix for examples.)
What thought has been playing on repeat today?
How are my feelings expressing themselves through my thoughts?
How did I talk myself into that bite/snack/binge?

Step 2: Name

Naming is simple. You're going to call what you notice *fruitful* or *not fruitful* based on the fruit of the Spirit (Gal. 5:19–23), which we've been exploring together throughout this journey, as well as Philippians 4:8:

> Finally, brothers, whatever is true, whatever is honorable, whatever is just, whatever is pure, whatever is lovely, whatever is commendable, if there is any excellence, if there is anything worthy of praise, think about these things.

True, notable, right, pure, lovely, admirable, excellent, and praiseworthy thoughts are fruitful thoughts and beliefs.

Step 3: Renew

Now that you've noticed and named, it's time to renew. This step may be as quick or study-soaked as you desire. For example, you may notice a sabotaging thought and have a quick rewrite that resonates with you.

"I already ate one—I'll start tomorrow," is quickly replaced with "My chance to make a different choice is *now*." However, a deep-seated limiting belief, such as "I'll never be good enough," will require some prayerful and purposeful time in God's Word, looking up verses about who you are in Christ. In fact, if you come across a sticky belief that won't let you go, consider pausing in this chapter to do some concentrated study, allowing the Holy Spirit to heal your heart and mind.

To help you compose a renewed thought, consider asking yourself the following questions:

Is this 100 percent, beyond a shadow of a doubt, true?
What evidence is there to support this thought?
Is there an alternative way to look at this?

What does Scripture say about this?

What would Jesus say about this?

Pray and ask the Holy Spirit to direct you to Scripture. Spend some time looking up Scriptures related to your thoughts, or put on your friend hat and counsel yourself like you would a loved one. Then give yourself plenty of time to mold a renewed thought, a rebuttal to the old thought or belief, that truly resonates with you.

Here are a few examples to get your creative juices flowing.

Fruit-Filled Journaling

Notice	Name	Renew
Jot down the thought.	Is the thought fruitful or not fruitful?	What is the new truth? What does God's Word say about this thought?
"I'm not making progress, so I may as well eat this."	not fruitful	"The reason I am not making progress is because I make all these little compromises that add up! That's okay; today I can do something different and wait to eat until I'm hungry."
"It's been a hard day; I deserve a sweet treat."	not fruitful	"Hard days are *hard*. What I need is permission to rest, have self-compassion, and eat a nutritious meal."
"I'll never be successful."	not fruitful	"Only God knows the future. The only way to ensure failure is to stop trying. I am going to keep showing up, despite my doubts, to see what God will do!"
"I can't control myself around food."	not fruitful	"I have the Holy Spirit and the fruit of the Spirit in my life. I have made self-controlled choices in my eating before. I refuse to adopt this unhelpful belief."

While these examples may or may not resonate with you, do you feel the difference between the first and the third column? One speaks destruction while the other speaks life. When you begin to encourage yourself in the Lord, you exchange your horizontal focus for a vertical one.

PERSONALIZE YOUR HABIT

Ready to think higher? You'll start Fruit-Filled Journaling by choosing a designated time to practice your new habit. It's important to begin with an intentional but flexible routine so that you can become proficient in this process. Then, in time, you'll find yourself transforming your thoughts in the moment (Thank you, Jesus!) and using a journal, as needed, for those sticky statements you want to tackle over time. But for now, find a space and place to ensure you get into a groove.

Let's review the three steps and pick your plan.

Step 1: Notice. How are you going to record those limiting beliefs and sabotaging thoughts? You may want to tuck a small journal or 3×5 card in your purse or use your notes app. When you have a convenient way to jot down your thoughts, you'll be able to collect them on the go. Of course, you don't have to write them down immediately (or even write them all), but a scribbled piece of paper is easier to manage than a scattered mind. Ultimately, do what feels sustainable and effective and kick any unrealistic expectations to the curb.

Step 2: Name. Call those thoughts *fruitful* or *not fruitful*. You can do this on the fly or when you sit down to renew. Easy, right?

Step 3: Renew. Here's where the miraculous is made known. As you renew your thoughts, you'll be talking to God, searching the Scriptures, meditating on his truth, and creating shiny new neural pathways in your brain. Simply questioning those old, worn-out lies can begin to weaken the hold they have on you and create a more peaceful mental and emotional space. How will practicing step 3 be most beneficial for you? You may want to look for a pocket of time every day or a few times a week to review and renew your list. If you're looking for a Bible study, a topical study specific to your thinking patterns would be an excellent way to engage with God's Word.

Fruit-Filled Journaling Tips

Look for Patterns

While our minds may feel chaotic, our thoughts tend to follow common paths or patterns. For example, you may notice that yesterday you were irritated at yourself when you missed an important phone call, frustrated because you forgot the laundry in the washer until it was musty, and scolded yourself after an impulsive candy bar purchase.

Three different situations with varying thoughts, and all are rooted in self-criticism.

Having spotted this pattern, you can now look up Scriptures that speak to the nature of self-criticism and be reminded that we all fall short of the glory of God (Rom. 3:23) and that we're to stir one another up for love and good works (Heb. 10:24). You also remember that gentleness and patience are fruit of the Spirit. This may allow a single positive thought to remedy numerous unfruitful thoughts all at once: *Only God is perfect. Self-criticism will just keep me stuck. I'll show myself grace and move on to the next best thing.*

Watch Out for Self-Condemnation

As you begin to examine your thoughts, you may notice some struggles you didn't realize were there or see some patterns you're ready to let go of . . . yesterday. When this happens, you can lose patience with yourself, get frustrated, and replace old thoughts with new condemnations. Not helpful. Let's take a moment to differentiate between conviction and condemnation.

Conviction strengthens our relationship with God. While the correction may sting initially, this nudge to be more Christlike is followed with joy and excitement as we catch the vision of what a life enlightened with God's Word will look like.

Condemnation causes us to feel separated from God as it heaps on guilt and shame, making us think we need to fix our problems on our own. But God did everything he could to adopt us into his family so that we may call to him, "Abba! Father!" (Rom. 8:14–15), and so that we may run boldly to him in our times of need (Heb. 4:15–16).

Guard your heart from condemnation and replace it with the reality about *who you are* in Christ.

Let Go of Perfectionism

As you work on creating fruitful rebuttals for your unfruitful thoughts, you may find yourself looking for just the right replacement thought—the one you believe will "change everything." And while it's amazing when the Lord gives us a word from his lips to our hearts, any thought rooted in the Word will help. Let's stop making it about our performance and focus on our Father.

Do your best and let go of the rest. Be okay with the learning curve. Old thinking patterns don't unravel on their own, but even a halfhearted response does more for your food freedom than letting old thoughts run wild.

Embrace the journey, celebrate the wins, and let the setbacks teach you how to bounce back more quickly so that your mind can be a blessing.

When Your Mind Is Your Ally

My heart sank when I looked at the clock and remembered my 2:00 dentist appointment. It was 1:45 and I'd never make it there on time. I picked up the phone to let the dental office know that I wasn't going to make it. I offered to pay the missed appointment fee, but they understood; things like this happen. I moved on with my day, appreciative for the grace and the reminder to keep an eye on my calendar.

The unexpected free time turned out to be a blessing, as the afternoon unfolded like a relentless game of whack-a-mole, with one issue popping up after another. *Take it one step at a time,* I assured myself. *Nothing is urgent, and what is important always gets done.* By the time I walked through my door at the end of the day, I was exhausted and hungry, and there was much to be done. *First, a moment to breathe,* I decided. I brewed a soothing cup of tea, sliced an apple, and then settled into my cozy corner of the couch. As I snacked and sipped, I leisurely flipped through a catalog that had arrived in the mail, allowing myself to unwind. After about fifteen minutes, I felt rejuvenated enough to start dinner prep. I put on my favorite podcast and listened to it as I cooked, waiting for my husband to come home.

After dinner and cleanup, I usually take a walk, but this time I felt ready to call it a night. Then I reminded myself that I'm someone who takes a walk after dinner because moving makes me feel good. I hooked the dog onto her leash, walked my neighborhood loop, and came home feeling refreshed.

Ah, the beauty of Fruitful Habits.

When it was finally time to wind down, I didn't feel the pull of the fridge like I used to. There were no negative thoughts to drown out or ravenous emotions to soothe. Whatever was left from the day felt manageable, and I knew a good night's sleep was what I needed most.

This was just an ordinary day, full of its own trouble, just like the day I told you about at the beginning of this chapter. The difference was the story I was telling myself. I believed that the Lord had gone ahead of me and was behind me (Ps. 139:5), that he was my portion (Lam. 3:24), and that he was working on my behalf (Rom. 8:28).

And I did my best to live like it.

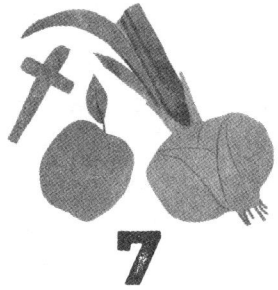

THE ONLY TWO THINGS
YOU CAN CHANGE

Trust in the LORD *with all your heart, and do not lean on your own understanding. In all your ways acknowledge him, and he will make straight your paths.*

Proverbs 3:5–6

Sarah stood in the middle of her kitchen, staring at a pile of unfamiliar ingredients and unusual spices, a new recipe book propped open on the counter next to the brand-new ultra-accurate digital food scale she'd purchased yesterday. It was the beginning of her journey toward healthier eating. But she was off to a rocky start. Just finding what she needed to get started had been stressful and expensive. Skimming the recipe she'd chosen, she was overwhelmed by its detailed steps and instructions. First, she needed to chiffonade the kale and rinse the quinoa. She didn't know how to do or even *say* that.

As she began weighing and measuring each item, trying to calculate her macros, her family wandered into the kitchen, eyeing the unfamiliar foods with suspicion. Her husband raised an eyebrow at the leafy greens, and her kids poked at the quinoa as if it might come alive. The atmosphere thickened with their skepticism, making Sarah's task even more daunting.

Halfway through the preparation, her youngest complained, "Why can't we just have spaghetti?" Her husband, sensing the rising tension and Sarah's growing frustration, gently suggested, "Maybe we could just order pizza tonight?"

At that moment, overwhelmed by the challenge of balancing new eating habits with her family's preferences for the familiar and the complicated details of the recipe, Sarah felt her resolve crumble. The thought of continuing was just too much.

With a sigh of disappointment, she closed the cookbook, turned off the stove, and picked up her phone to order a meal she knew would bring smiles rather than scowls to the dinner table. As she dialed, Sarah looked at the unused ingredients, now likely to go to waste.

This wasn't the first time her good intentions had ended up sidelined by the overwhelming task of overhauling her diet overnight. It was clear she needed a simpler, more gradual approach to healthy eating—one that wouldn't leave her feeling defeated before she even began.

Whoever thought something as natural as eating could be so complicated?

Whether you have a big family or not, I bet you can relate to how overwhelming idealistic eating can be. It seems to be that when it comes to changing our diets, we want to overhaul everything, all at once. New recipes, new foods, new cooking methods, new apps, new portion sizes, new "good" foods, new "bad" foods. Then we get upset with ourselves when we can't seem to manage all the newness.

But you and I understand from past experiences that transformative learning doesn't take place overnight. You knew you wouldn't excel at piano, tennis, or French right away, right? But you gave yourself the grace and space to practice and improve, and you did.

As we've discussed, the same principles apply to eating. Grace and space give us the breathing room to get better. What would've happened if Sarah had just been excited that she wanted to prepare a nourishing meal but didn't get bogged down in the details? She probably would've eaten a pretty nutritious dinner, felt satisfied, and been one step closer to restoring her relationship with food.

Eating should not be complicated, and neither should eating well. At the end of the day, every "healthy eating" plan can only do two things: change *how much* you eat (quantity) or *what* you eat (quality). That's it. But rather than embracing the simplicity of these two things, diet makers create endless rules and restrictions that make eating feel confusing, overwhelming, and impossible to maintain.

I'm going to show you how to focus in by panning out. But first, let's remind ourselves of the importance of small, sustainable habits and firm up our foundation.

No More "Go Big or Go Home"

Our lives are entrenched with more all-or-nothing thinking than we probably realize. The admonition to push hard or else it doesn't matter is plastered on gym walls, locker rooms, executive offices, and maybe even the backdrop of your mind.

But what if, as you discovered in chapter 4, "Uncover the Goals That Motivate You," your definition of success has nothing to do with leaving it all on the field? What if you desire quality of life more than perfect adherence to the latest food plan?

What if all this dietary micromanaging is too much for you because . . . it *is* too much? When we're overly concerned with refining dietary details, calculating carbs, or analyzing nutrition labels, we tend to overlook the big-picture habits that hinder our goals: poor food quality or excess food quantity.

Think about it: Every diet plan you've been on has addressed one or both of these areas. Some in more obvious ways, such as weighing, measuring, or color-coded food lists. Others in more subtle ways, such as eating when you're hungry and stopping when you're full. Ultimately, all of these plans change the type or amount of food you eat—probably in a bunch of different ways and all at once.

But in our journey together, you'll continue to take one step at a time, giving yourself the grace and space you need to adopt new habits at your own pace. When you do this, your habits become new routines, making them easy to do even on a hard day. With a big-picture perspective and a small-habit approach, you'll be pleased to see how many of those nagging details will resolve themselves.

In this chapter, you'll be introduced to the concepts related to food quality and food quantity. Then, in the following two chapters, you'll learn about the importance of satisfying nutrition as well as how to reconnect to your hunger and fullness cues. Together, these three chapters will provide a benchmark of healthy eating habits—all while preserving your peace.

But before we move on, let's do a check-in on your journey so far. You began by building a solid foundation of grace and gratitude, confronting all-or-nothing thinking and negative body image right off the bat. Then you explored your deeper motivations, aligned them with your values, and embraced fruit-filled habits and beliefs. These steps are essential before diving into the specifics of how to eat; they ensure that the peace you've gained now serves as your guide.

So, how do you shift into a more food-centric focus without losing your Jesus-first focus? You preserve the habits and mindsets you began with. Specifically:

- **In chapter 1, you learned to maintain a mindset of gratitude.** As you begin to change a little more of "how you eat," remember to start from a place of thankfulness—acknowledging all you have and how far you've come. Your Grow in Gratitude habit will help you keep your eyes on the Lord and on the purpose behind your efforts.

- **In chapter 2, you discovered how to watch out for all-or-nothing thinking.** Because our histories make us prone to turning just about any eating change into a "diet," stay watchful for this detrimental mindset. Instead, aim to be 1 percent better today and let go of the rest. You may want to frame your Quality or Quantity habit as a Seed of Self-Control to help you keep a faith-first approach.

- **In chapter 3, you saw how to keep the scale in its proper place.** If you're aiming to lose weight, you may be tempted to measure your "success" by the scale. But it's crucial to guard your heart. Don't let your mind linger there—it will only reignite the diet mentality! Lasting weight loss requires consistency and sustainability, which are found when your motivation is deeply connected to your personal goals and values. The Mind-Body Scan habit can help you observe if changes in your food quality or quantity start to bring your hunger and fullness cues to life.

If any of these habits have slipped and you feel it's time for a tune-up, you may want to take a few days to reestablish your practice before moving on. Don't give an *inch* of what you've gained back to the enemy; only be satisfied with claiming even more territory.

Habits 7 and 8: Food Quality or Food Quantity

As we've discussed, when it comes to improving your eating habits, you can only change two things: *what* or *how much* you eat.

Diets bog you down with directions and details, but your new path will guide you to prayerfully choose a change that is doable, sustainable, appealing, and effective.

In this chapter, you'll focus on quality *or* quantity. Not both at once. Just one.

"Why's that?" you ask. Because trying to do too much will only dilute your efforts and make you less effective. More is not better if more is not attainable.

After you've practiced your Quality or Quantity habit, you may want to spend some extra time in this chapter implementing the other option. Or you can keep moving forward and revisit these habits later in chapter 11, "How to Stay Free."

But which should you choose? Don't worry, I've got you covered. Below is a brief quiz designed to help you decide which path is best for you. Then we'll dive into the details of each option. Regardless of your quiz results, it's a good idea to review both sections. This way, you can make a well-informed choice and confirm which approach you'll begin with.

Read each line and choose the answer that best suits you.

Quality OR Quantity?

Quality		Quantity
I'd rather eat a larger portion of lighter food.	OR	I'd rather eat a smaller portion of rich food.
I prefer fruits and veggies.	OR	I prefer cheese and nuts.
I like to cook.	OR	I'd rather eat out.
I like the idea of choosing higher-quality food.	OR	I'm not quite ready to change what I eat.
I really want to eat healthier food!	OR	I really want to reconnect with my hunger and fullness signals!
I'm not quite ready to think about how much I eat.	OR	I like the idea of adjusting my portion sizes.

If you chose more options on the left-hand side, the Food Quality path may be the simpler place for you to start. If you chose more options on the right-hand side, the Food Quantity path may be where you begin.

Still not sure? Start with the quality path to ensure your meals are satisfying, and then you can adjust your portion sizes later. If you need additional direction or support, consider consulting with a registered dietitian for guidance on your food quality and quantity.

HABIT 7: FOOD QUALITY

Welcome to the Food Quality path, where your habit is to slowly change *what* you eat.

Throughout the book, we've emphasized that food is simply "just food." Donuts aren't "bad" and broccoli isn't "righteous." God is far more concerned with the state of our hearts than the contents of our bellies.

However, there are some foods that fuel and nourish our bodies better than others—these are whole, unprocessed foods. Such "real food" is incredible; it's high in fiber and loaded with vitamins, minerals, and antioxidants that provide the human body with the synergistic nutrients it needs to thrive. Whole foods are foods closest to their God-given state, such as fruits, vegetables, beans, grains, nuts, seeds, meat, fish, and eggs. We'll dive more into nutrition in chapter 8, but for now let's agree that eating more of what God made is a good thing!

The Whole Foods Continuum

I bet you're wondering if your favorite yogurt or whole wheat pasta are considered whole foods. To answer these questions, first stop thinking about food as existing in separate columns such as red (don't eat), yellow (avoid), and green (eat)—and start to imagine them along a continuum. Picture a horizontal line: On the left is where you are today, and on the right is you eating more whole foods. Along the way, there are as many steps as you want or need to take. To start your walk on the Food Quality path, you'll simply take one step along the continuum. Let's look at a few examples.

Suppose you often rely on frozen meals. To walk the quality path, you could increase your whole-food consumption by choosing a different frozen meal that has fewer additives, add a side of veggies, or try cooking a meal at home once or twice a week. Or maybe your lunch and dinner are pretty dialed in, but your breakfast could use some work. You can look for delicious ways to upgrade your morning meal, one step at a time.

Notice the beauty of embracing progress over perfection. As your meals become more nourishing, you'll begin to genuinely appreciate sweets and treats, knowing your daily habits support your long-term health.

What might that look like?

- Add a serving of produce to one or more of your daily meals.
- Aim for approximately one-fourth or one-half of your plate to be whole foods.
- Upgrade your breakfast, lunch, dinner, or snack, which may look like trying one of these simple swaps:

Replace sweetened instant oatmeal with rolled oats with honey and fruit.

Replace sweetened yogurt with plain Greek yogurt with maple syrup and fruit.

Instead of sweetened breakfast cereal, choose a cereal with less sugar.

Replace a frozen breakfast sandwich with eggs and sprouted grain toast.

For frozen meals, look for alternate brands with more natural ingredients or try a new recipe at home.

For fast-food meals, swap part of your meal for a side salad or look for a restaurant that offers healthier options.

Replace white pasta with whole wheat or lentil pasta.

Replace white bread with whole grain bread or a high fiber wrap.

Instead of a granola bar, have a serving of nuts and fruit.

For chips and pretzels, look for alternate brands with more natural ingredients.

THE CONTINUUM OF THE QUALITY PATH

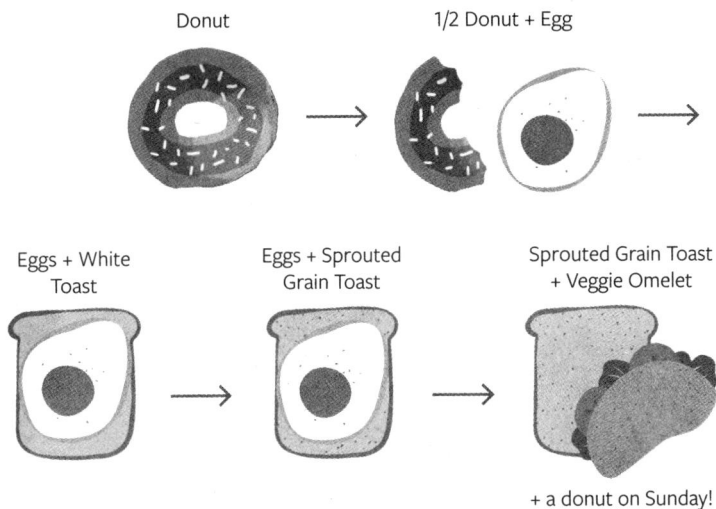

Donut   1/2 Donut + Egg

Eggs + White   Eggs + Sprouted   Sprouted Grain Toast
Toast   Grain Toast   + Veggie Omelet

+ a donut on Sunday!

Wisdom is revealed in choosing achievable goals. You're simply looking for the next step along the continuum.

"But what if I already eat 'healthy'?" you may ask.

If your meals are mostly whole foods, then switch to the quantity path. However, if you struggle with secret eating—eating well in front of others but then bingeing on processed foods when you're alone— then the best way to improve your overall food quality is to start including some of those "forbidden foods" into your regular meals.

For example, if you have a salad with chicken for lunch but end up raiding the pantry for chips and cookies at 3:00 p.m., try having a serving of chips with your lunch and a cookie after dinner. It may feel uncomfortable at first, but bringing your eating into the light and enjoying what you consume is a crucial step in finding food freedom.

Personalize Your Quality Habit

Now it's time to get specific. How do you envision Food Quality weaving through your life? What are the specific ways you can improve your food quality without uprooting your food freedom? If you're not entirely sure where to get started, now's a great time to freshen up your Simply Plan Ahead habit from chapter 4 and get those whole foods into your pantry.

Once you've chosen your Food Quality habit, add a reminder to put the foods you want to include on your grocery list. Got it? You'll practice it for the next week (or longer, if you want to take time to really let it sink in). Be sure to use your free habit tracker and follow along with the included Scripture writing pages to keep your habit and Jesus-first focus front and center.

HABIT 8: FOOD QUANTITY

Welcome to Food Quantity, where your habit is to slightly adjust *how much* you eat. I needed this path when I had been trying to follow the "eat when you're hungry and stop when you're full" approach but dieting had drowned out any semblance of a reliable body signal. Mostly, I'd plow right past full because when I did try to stop eating sooner, I'd undershoot and be too hungry too soon, and then overeat in response. It drove me to distraction!

While the goal is to be guided by the body's cues, which we'll explore in chapter 9, it's often easier to let these signals naturally emerge rather than actively search for them. And the simplest way to do that is to purposefully adjust how much you eat—not a lot, but a little at a time. This could look like reducing your portion sizes at one or more meals, tapering off any unneeded snacks, or making your meals more substantial if you tend to undereat at meals and then graze or binge later.

Personalize Your Quantity Habit

Before you choose your specific Food Quantity habit, it's essential to consider whether your portions or meal frequency might need to increase or decrease. Often we associate adjusting portions with eating less, but for some, the challenge is eating *enough* at meals and scheduled snacks to fully nourish the body. Feeling full, satisfied, and energized between meals is key to achieving food freedom.

Take a moment to reflect on your experiences with these simple questions:

How do you feel after you eat?

If you feel sluggish or uncomfortable and rarely feel hunger before your next meal, you'll likely benefit from eating a bit less.

If you're still preoccupied with food, grazing between meals, or overly hungry before your next meal, you'll likely benefit from making your meals more substantial.

How often do you eat?

Do you graze between meals and snacks? You might benefit from shifting those extra bites to mealtimes, allowing you to walk away fully satisfied.

Do you let yourself get too hungry? If you go more than five hours between meals, try adding a snack. If it's less than three hours, consider increasing the portion size at your previous meal.

Reflect and Adjust

Your answers can help you determine whether your Food Quantity habit might involve scaling back, eating a bit more to find satisfaction, or shifting extra BLTs (bites, licks, and tastes) to your meals.

In chapter 8, we'll explore practical tools like portion guides and macronutrient balance to help you fine-tune your meals. For now, focus on observing how much you eat and making choices that feel doable, sustainable, and aligned with your needs.

Once you've reflected on your needs, here are a few ways to begin walking the quantity path:

- **Feeling too full after meals?** Try serving yourself three bites less or leaving three bites on your plate to create a comfortable level of fullness.
- **Snacking out of habit instead of hunger?** Taper back or skip the snack if your next meal is near, allowing your hunger to build naturally.
- **Sow a Seed of Self-Control.** "Fast" during times when you tend to graze mindlessly, such as during dinner prep or while watching TV, and redirect your focus to a satisfying mealtime instead.
- **Gather your grazing.** If you tend to undereat at meals but find yourself nibbling throughout the day, shift those extra bites to your meals to feel satisfied and reduce the need to snack later.

These habits can help you discover how varying portion sizes and timing work best for you. Pay attention to the feedback your body gives and adjust as needed. For example, consider your body's cues regarding your afternoon snack:

- **Pleasantly hungry for dinner?** Your snack size was just right.
- **Not hungry at all at dinnertime?** You might not need a snack.
- **Too hungry at dinnertime?** You may have cut back too much.

The goal of Food Quantity is to gently adjust your portions or meal timing until you're eating the right amount for your needs—leaving you satisfied, nourished, and free from preoccupation with food.

Again, adjusting your food quantity is not an admonition to undereat. Undereating is never good for you, and it will only lead to overeating later—likely in greater quantity and lesser quality than if you'd simply enjoyed a satisfying meal.

If you're eating too little at meals and end up grazing or overeating, consider planning your day around three meals and one or two snacks. Find a consistent routine before adjusting portion sizes.

Remember, this is a process of learning and adjusting (and it's kind of like learning a new language), so please show yourself grace.

When Clarity Replaces Confusion

You've moved from the confusion of contradictory diet rules to the clarity of a simpler focus, and you're ready to gently adjust your food quality or quantity. These flexible habits will allow you to find the types and amounts of food that work best for *your* unique body. Pretty amazing, right?

You may want to camp out in this chapter, giving yourself an opportunity to practice both Food Quality and Food Quantity, or you may be ready to venture into the next two nutrition-centric chapters. Either way, here's a quick reminder to keep your foundation strong by practicing grace and gratitude and defeating that all-or-nothing thinking. Avoid the distraction caused by getting overly focused on food and remain clear: You are not the primary source of your strength in this journey to food freedom. It's not about the details of what you eat but about the desires of your heart.

Keep your eyes locked on Jesus, continue asking the Holy Spirit for wisdom, and you will stand strong.

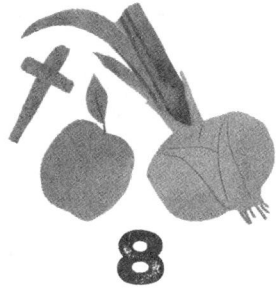

8

NUTRITION MADE SIMPLE

So, whether you eat or drink, or whatever you do, do all to the glory of God.

1 Corinthians 10:31

Why do we feel like we need to fit into a food box?

I'm not talking about takeout. I'm referring to the idea that our eating should be compartmentalized, labeled, or defined. Maybe we're low-carb, keto, vegetarian, or an intuitive eater. We're following *this* plan or reading *that* book.

We're dieting, or . . . we're not.

We're eating healthy, or . . . we're not.

But what if all these labels and ideals are distancing us from discovering our own individualized nutrition?

What if *your* best way of eating, the one where you leave the table full, satisfied, energized, and able to move on without thinking about food, doesn't fit in a diet box—or it hops from one box to another, based on your day? What if loosening every label and giving yourself permission to uncover what works best for you would finally lead to discovering what does? What if eating meals that satisfied you resolved some of those nagging cravings?

In this chapter, you're going to learn about the marvel of *satisfaction* and how to eat in a way that satisfies you, fully.

It's Not About Food, but Food Matters

We've already learned how our struggles with eating are about so much more than food. In the past, it may have seemed like food was our primary remedy for almost any challenge.

Have a bad day? Seek solace in a treat.

Have a bad breakout? Surely something we ate is to blame.

In those scenarios, food is the problem *and* the solution. Once we can see how our thoughts, feelings, and emotions are the driving force behind many of our food struggles, we can discover how to meet our true needs, one step at a time.

But what we eat still matters as it impacts how we feel—mentally, physically, and emotionally. Yes, nutrition is part of it, but it's about so much more than vitamins and minerals. It's about satisfaction. Have you ever . . .

Eaten a whole box of "healthy" cookies but still craved a home-made one? You were missing mental satisfaction.

Devoured a stack of pancakes only to feel the urge to eat an hour later? You were missing physical satisfaction.

Ate to soothe emotional pain but then couldn't stop eating? You were missing emotional satisfaction.

When we eat without the awareness of what will satisfy us, food will occupy more space than we'd like to give it.

To clearly discern our physical satisfaction, we ought to be spiritually satisfied. Because nothing but Jesus can fill us when our spirit is hungry. We were *created* to be satisfied.

Our God is a God of more than enough. But the fullness he provides isn't meant to overstuff us; it's meant to overflow from us (2 Cor. 9:8). The purpose of our healing, through our relationship with Jesus Christ, is so that we can help others do the same. Of course, this takes time, but you're already making progress in renewing your mind and learning how to satisfy your deepest needs by addressing the root cause of your food struggles.

The Lord created us to be satisfied in *every* area of life. This satisfaction doesn't always look the way we expect, as our hearts can be content and peaceful, trusting in God's care and provision, even in times of "lack" (Phil. 4:11–13). True satisfaction is a place of contentment, a happy sigh of "God is enough."

Overeating pushes past this point because a discontented heart can never be truly satiated by food. Eating can't fill the void or heal emotional wounds. When we learn to separate the call for rest, prayer, or a good cry from the call for food, we'll have realistic expectations of our meals that they can finally fulfill.

Conversely, eating *is* about more than physical hunger—it's intertwined with our mental and emotional well-being too. For example, we all have thoughts and feelings about what we eat—our likes, pleasant food memories, or joy in fellowship. These are all healthy ways to weave food into our already full lives, which is quite different from using food to cope with our emotions.

When your spirit is being fed and your emotions have a voice, it becomes easier to find mental satisfaction in your eating. And mental satisfaction may be the missing piece (or peace) in your meals.

Mental Satisfaction

Have you ever considered the role mental satisfaction plays in being content and satiated with your meal? Mental satisfaction has more to do with your thoughts and feelings regarding your food choices than the actual amount or type of food you eat. It involves considering what foods you truly want, hearing yourself, and making choices that marry your wants with wisdom.

Think about a time when you ate something you thought you "should" have, based on your internal food rules. As you crammed mounds of "healthy" food into your mouth, you were probably eyeing everyone else's plates, wishing they were yours. If you're anything like me, you got up from the table irritated and disappointed, only to raid the kitchen after everyone else had gone to bed, still trying to satisfy those lingering cravings (goodbye, box of cereal).

On the other hand, there may have been times when you ate with abandon, all in the name of "eating what you want," only to walk away overfull and unhappy (unsatisfied) with your choices.

As you can see, mental satisfaction is about making choices that feel right for you based on what you like and what matters to you. It's about tuning in to your own preferences and values when deciding what to eat. So, how does one achieve mental satisfaction at meals? Here are three things to consider.

Step 1: Honor Your Preferences

Ask yourself: **What do I *truly* want?** As we discussed in chapter 4, you have eating preferences. You may be the only one in your family who likes sushi or the only one who doesn't. When you honor those preferences and choose what you truly enjoy rather than what you think you *should* or *shouldn't* have, you'll ditch deprivation because you're eating what you genuinely want. Over time, this will likely become a mix of fun and nutritious foods.

Step 2: Notice Your Mindset

Ask yourself: **How are my feelings affecting my wants?** If the thought of eating "what you want" scares you, it's likely because you're recalling your emotional cravings—those strong urges at the end of a stressful day or the all-or-nothing thinking that drives you to eat. When you eat to soothe your emotions, you often find yourself mentally unsatisfied because you're applying the wrong medicine to your wounds. That's why noticing your thoughts is so helpful. The more you pay attention to your mindset, the easier it becomes to make mindful choices.

Yes, there will still be times when you choose to eat emotionally, and that's okay. It happens. However, when you're more aware of the reasons you turn to food and its outcomes, you'll be less drawn to this pseudo-solution next time.

Step 3: Respect Your Values

Ask yourself: **What choice will best reflect what I value?** To feel truly mentally satisfied with your meals, you'll want them to have *some* alignment with your values. Why just "some" and not "complete"? Because perfect alignment between your values and your eating isn't necessary or realistic. However, aligning with your values as much as you can is still important. For example:

- *Do you value family time?* Avoiding a family event because of a food rule might feel pretty icky.
- *Do you value health?* Completely ignoring your desire to eat well could leave you feeling pretty icky too.
- *Do you value faith?* Ignoring the guidance of the Holy Spirit regarding food will likely feel—you guessed it—pretty icky.

Regularly ignoring what truly matters to you can create feelings of misalignment, which can be quite uncomfortable and may lead to emotional overeating.

Satisfaction is about more than how much you eat. Of course, these steps are not intended to be a pre-meal interrogation. However, if you notice that you're feeling unsure about your food choices, taking a moment to review these questions before you eat can help you identify a few thoughts worth exploring through your Fruit-Filled Journaling habit.

Physical Satisfaction

You're not short on nutritional knowledge—you know that veggies are better for you than cupcakes—but the real shift in eating habits externally happens when you change your relationship with food internally. As you continue to renew your mind, you'll become even better equipped to make choices that come from a place of spiritual health and self-care. This is the foundation we'll continue to build upon as we explore physical satisfaction, nutrition, and macronutrients.

Your habit for this chapter is Balance Out Your Plate, an intentional shift toward meals that best meet your nutritional needs. We'll dive into the details later, but for now it's important for you to know that a balanced plate is one that has a showing of each of the three macronutrients: protein, carbohydrates, and fat. I'm sure you've heard of them (wink, wink). While many diets restrict or eliminate certain macronutrients, each one offers unique nutritional and satiety benefits. We're going to learn (or relearn) about these nutrients from a satisfaction standpoint—how each one serves you so that *you* can serve well.

While the majority of foods contain a mix of protein, carbohydrates, and fat, many contain predominantly one. Whether you've spent time meticulously tracking each gram or haven't given the "big three" much thought, I'm going to ask you to set aside your previous experiences and be open to a new, freeing, empowering perspective.

In the following section, we'll explore each macronutrient through the lens of its function and its fruit. This perspective will help you create balance—meals that satisfy you both mentally and physically—so you can move on and stop overthinking what to eat.

Protein Made Simple

Protein is satisfying. High-protein foods include meat, fish, eggs, dairy, and tofu. For non-meat eaters, legumes (beans) are also counted as protein. For those who do eat meat, legumes may be considered carbohydrates, which we'll cover in the next section.

The amazing thing about protein is how satiating it can be—filling us up during a meal but also keeping us fuller longer, thanks to its slow rate of digestion.

Most meat eaters easily meet their minimum protein requirements. However, eating a bit more than the recommended daily allowance (RDA) can offer several benefits beyond weight loss. Protein plays a vital role in the body: It helps maintain lean body mass, supports tissue healing, regulates blood sugar and hormones, and serves as a precursor for neurotransmitters that impact mood and mental clarity. These benefits make protein an essential part of a balanced diet for everyone.

Many diets emphasize lean proteins because these typically contain less fat and fewer calories, making it harder to overeat ("I'll take a third helping of boiled chicken breast," said no one, ever). But there's no need to overthink what type of protein you choose.

A QUICK NOTE FOR THOSE WITH FOOD RESTRICTIONS

If you have specific dietary restrictions due to celiac disease, allergies, or other medical needs that impact your nutrition, these principles can still apply. However, it may be wise to consult a qualified healthcare provider or registered dietitian to help you adapt these habits safely and confidently to support your well-being. The key is to honor your body's requirements by choosing safe and nourishing foods that fit within your unique needs. For example, if you need to be gluten-free, focus on gluten-free whole grains or starchy vegetables for carbohydrates.

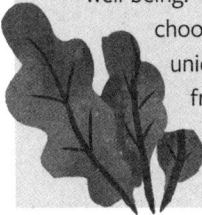

Fattier cuts of meat can be just as nutritious, are often more satisfying, and can even count as the fat portion of your meal.

By focusing on the many roles protein plays in your health, you can begin to see it as more than just a "diet food." It's a vital building block for a strong, well-functioning body and a key to feeling energized and satisfied.

Carbohydrates Made Simple

Carbohydrates, aka "carbs," are grains, root vegetables, fruits, and legumes for those who eat meat. In this section, we'll explore three types of carbohydrates and their unique benefits.

1. Starchy Carbs

Starchy carbs are energizing. Starchy carbs include grains, potatoes, winter squash, and beans. These fiber-filled foods provide sustained energy and hydration (carbo-hydrate), helping to keep you full while nourishing your gut microbiome. Though they're higher in calories than fibrous carbs, they offer greater energy and satisfaction. For example, while a sweet potato (a starchy carb) has more calories than broccoli (a fibrous carb), it will keep you fuller for longer and provide the fuel you need to stay active.

If you've been trying to eat low-carb, adding starchy carbs to your plate can make you feel uneasy. But if you have nagging

SATISFYING MEAL TIP

Most meals will benefit from a palm-sized portion of protein.

If you jumped on the low-carb bandwagon, it's important to be aware that you *can* overeat protein. If you're regularly consuming a large portion (over 30 grams) at meals, you may benefit from paring back just a bit and making room for some other foods.

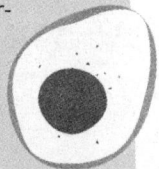

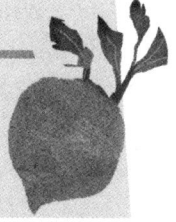

cravings, low energy, poor workout recovery, or unrestful sleep, the addition of starchy carbs may help alleviate some of those symptoms. Just be sure to add them gradually to give your body time to adjust.

If you're active or athletic, you may need more carbohydrates, so feel free to try larger portions. If you're less active, you'll probably need smaller amounts. However, make sure to include some starchy carbs in your meals regardless of your activity level.

2. Fibrous Carbs

Fibrous carbs are filling. Fibrous carbs are fruits and most vegetables. Thanks to their high fiber and water content, fibrous carbs help you feel full with fewer calories. They're also packed with micronutrients and antioxidants that support your overall health. However, balance is key. Skip fibrous carbs and you might notice decreased immune function, slower digestion, and a lack of fullness at meals. Overdo them and you may experience digestive distress and premature satiety, leading to a lack of energy.

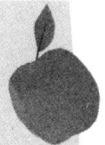

3. Processed Carbs

Processed carbs are fun. Processed carbs are packaged foods such as cookies, chips, candy, cakes, and crackers. When eaten independently, these carbohydrates provide a quick burst of energy that's often followed by a crash and cravings for more.

It's processed carbs that have cast a shadow over all carbohydrates. While you don't want to live exclusively on these foods, it's perfectly fine to include them on your plate.

How much and how often? Well, that's up to you. When it comes to health, less is best. Just remember, having some fun food on your plate is an essential part of mental satisfaction. If your "fun foods" include processed carbs, then planning them in will help you sustain your healthy habits long-term.

Fat Made Simple

Fats are sustaining. Fats are oils, butter, nuts, seeds, avocado, and some cheeses. As the most calorie-dense macronutrient, fats are digested slowly, keeping you fuller for longer between meals. Diets that are very low in fat will leave you in a near-constant state of dissatisfaction.

SATISFYING MEAL TIP

Pair processed carbs with protein, veggies, or a little fat to help regulate your blood sugar and increase satiety.

Adding these components slows down the absorption of processed carbs, keeping you fuller for longer and preventing energy crashes. For example, if you're craving a donut for breakfast but dislike the inevitable sugar crash an hour later, try pairing it with a hard-boiled egg for a boost of protein and fat to balance things out.

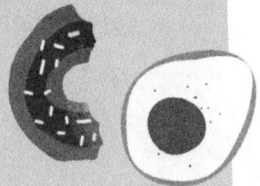

SATISFYING MEAL TIP ━━━━━━━━━━━━━━━

Most meals will benefit from one or two thumb-sized portions of fat.

You can adjust the fat content of your meals to influence how long you stay full. For example, I'll add two tablespoons of nut butter to my protein shake if I want it to keep me satiated for a while, or one tablespoon if my next meal is coming sooner.

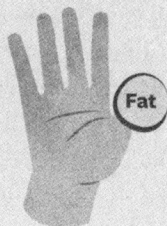

Because fats are rich and flavorful, they can be easy to overeat. They also enhance the taste of other foods, which can make those foods easier to overeat too. Interesting, right?

Due to its caloric density, you don't need a large portion of fat to feel satisfied. In fact, at some point, fat ceases to increase satiety. For example, let's say that you're having peanut butter toast for breakfast. One or two tablespoons of peanut butter feels great, but adding more would not increase your satisfaction in any remarkable way and would only add to your caloric bottom line.

Creating meals that are satisfying, energizing, filling, and sustaining is easy when you have a well-balanced plate. Of course, not every meal will be easy to classify. Perfection is not required—a simple shift into a more balanced, or balanced-out, plate is what we're looking for.

HABIT 9: BALANCE OUT YOUR PLATE ━━━━━━━━━━

Before now, you may have spent more time than you'd like to admit searching for the perfect diet or eating plan that would finally unlock your goals. I bet it feels great to have let go of that constant overanalyzing and overthinking. Now that you've started healing your relationship with food, I encourage you to see this next habit as a way to increase your self-care.

Food freedom is never about restriction.

Instead, we're discovering that making positive changes for our well-being is unlocking joy and peace—the new standard of fruitfulness we want our habits to meet. Our habit for this chapter, Balance Out Your Plate, was purposefully named to convey the aim for *more* balance, not perfect balance. Its primary goal is to help you feel energized and sustained by your meals and **not** for you to check off dietary boxes.

Do you remember the continuum of change we spoke about in the Quality Path section of the previous chapter? The idea is that we all have a starting point and a goal—a desired end result. Along this continuum of change, there are as many steps as we want or need to take.

To Balance Out Your Plate, you're going to take a moment to think about your most common meals and look at each of the three macronutrients.

It's as simple as:

> **Protein** ✓
> **Carbohydrate** ✓
> **Fat** ✓

If you notice that one macronutrient is either overrepresented or missing, consider how you can adjust your meal to make it more balanced. Often, this habit will be a subtle shift of doing a bit less of one thing and a bit more of another.

Need some ideas? Here are a few examples.

Balance Out Breakfast:
- If you typically start your day with oatmeal and a banana, you're primarily consuming carbohydrates. Consider a smaller portion of oatmeal and add some nuts (fat) and Greek yogurt (protein).

- If you tend to have a pretty low-carb breakfast like eggs and bacon (protein and fat), introduce some carbohydrates with a serving of fruit or some sprouted grain toast.

Balance Out Lunch:

- If you're a sandwich gal, stack it high with protein and veggies and include a source of fat like cheese, avocado, or a bit of mayonnaise (there are some great avocado oil options).

- If you're a salad and chicken gal (fibrous carbs and protein), start by taking a peek at how many fats your salad has—dressing, cheese, nuts, and avocado can unbalance your plate. You may want to stick to one or two fat sources in reasonable portions. To incorporate more starchy carbs, add some beans or quinoa, or enjoy a side of fruit or whole grain crackers.

Balance Out Dinner:

- If your dinners are fairly carbohydrate-based, such as pasta, casseroles, or pizza, consider adding some protein and veggies to your recipe or serve a side salad that includes both.

- If you're a meat-and-potatoes person, you likely have protein, fat, and carbohydrates covered. Adding a side of veggies will further balance your plate and make your meal even more satisfying.

Balance Out Snacks:

- When it comes to snacks, the more balanced, the better. However, it can be challenging to have protein, carbohydrates, *and* fat at snack time when you're just a little hungry. In that case, shoot for two macros, if possible.

If you're already eating the big three pretty consistently at each of your meals, reference the Satisfying Meal Tip sidebars in this chapter to make the most of your plate. You may need more or less food, but this is a jumping-off point to help you find your best way of eating. Ultimately, you'll allow hunger and fullness to guide your portions, which we'll dive into in the next chapter.

Not every plate will look like the one in this illustration, and that's okay. Any shift toward a more satisfying meal is a good thing. There may be a morning when what you truly want is a carb-centric breakfast. Great—eat it and enjoy it! You may have a lunchtime meeting that runs over, and all you have is a bag of almonds in your purse. No problem—eat them and move on.

If your meal is less than ideal, it's not a big deal if you don't make it one. Be on the lookout for the diet mindset. Ditch perfectionism and allow what you've learned about balancing out your plate to help you navigate any residual cravings. For example, if you decide to have a fruit smoothie or even ice cream for lunch, savor it

A BALANCED-OUT PLATE

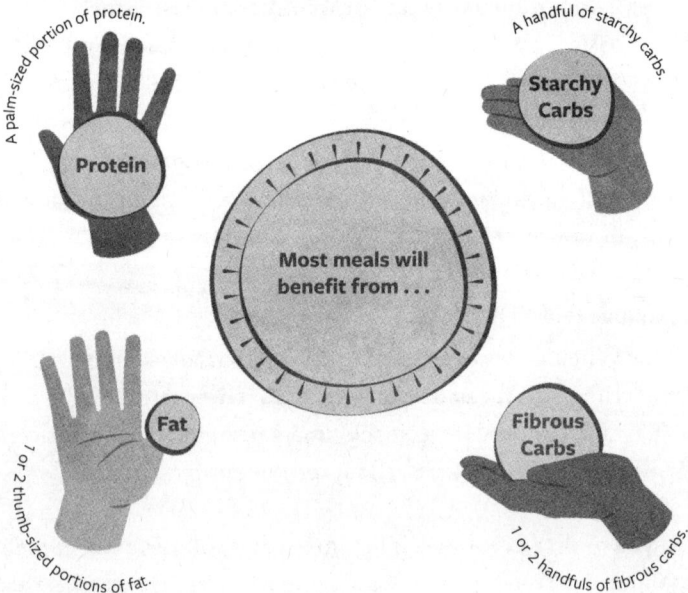

A palm-sized portion of protein.

Protein

A handful of starchy carbs.

Starchy Carbs

Most meals will benefit from . . .

Fat

1 or 2 thumb-sized portions of fat.

Fibrous Carbs

1 or 2 handfuls of fibrous carbs.

happily. Just be aware that you probably won't feel fully satisfied and will be craving sweets midday. Acknowledge those cravings as the ripple effect of an imbalanced meal, move on, and use them as a reminder to have a satisfying snack later. Remember, it's just one meal, and there are a thousand opportunities in the next 365 days to find that happy sigh of contentment.

PERSONALIZE YOUR HABIT

Now that we've seen macronutrients in a new light and painted a picture of a balanced-out plate, it's time for you to begin tweaking what you consume so food can start working *for* you, rather than the other way around.

When you think about your typical daily intake, is there one meal or one macro you'd like to start balancing out? Maybe breakfast would be the easiest entry point, you notice that your lunch is shy on protein, or you've been wanting to try some new dinner recipes. Pick one meal to start balancing out, make it your daily focus until it becomes your new normal, and then start to tweak another meal or snack.

Remember, this isn't about picking the perfect habit but working toward one that is doable, sustainable, appealing, and effective. The key to success is a bit of preplanning. When and where do you typically jot down your meals for the week? Where do you compile your grocery list? Now is a great time to add a note to Balance Out Your Plate in one or both of those places. This will serve as a reminder to plan and purchase what you need.

Okay, got your habit? You'll practice it for the next week (or longer, if you want to take time to really let it sink in). Be sure to use your free habit tracker and follow along with the included Scripture writing pages to keep your habit and Jesus-first focus front and center.

You, Satisfied

It's Saturday night, and you and your family are enjoying a scoop of ice cream at your favorite old-fashioned ice-cream shop. As you savor this time with your loved ones, you reflect on your past secret relationship with ice cream—so much eaten but never truly enjoyed. Now, butter pecan is a treat—in frequency, in taste, and, most of all, in your heart. There is no guilt or shame, just creamy deliciousness.

And the best part? You've just come from the pizza restaurant, where you had a slice and a half of cheese pizza and a side salad. You intentionally left enough room for ice cream because that feels good. There's no urgency to eat it all now; you know you'll be having pizza again next week. This is a joyful tradition with your family, and you are relishing every lick of it. Tomorrow, you'll get back to your normal routine, but Saturday nights are meant to be savored.

How did you find this fabulous relationship with food? You started by meeting your true needs first, in Christ—the ones that have nothing to do with food. This allowed you to finally discern how to eat in a way that feels good to you. Then you embraced the importance of satisfaction, understanding that nourishment is not about counting calories but about how food makes you feel, inside and out. You learned to fuel your body so that food could fuel your life, making your macros and meals work for you—not the other way around.

Now food is just one fun part of your life. It can't fix your problems, but it doesn't have to cause them either. Thank you, Jesus!

9

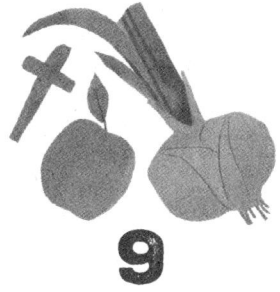

DECODING HUNGER AND FULLNESS

*Blessed are those who hunger and thirst for righteousness,
for they shall be satisfied.*

Matthew 5:6

"I think I'm full," you say in surprise, looking at the half sandwich still on your plate.

"Is that hunger?" you wonder, noticing it's almost time to start making dinner.

While hunger and fullness may have felt uncomfortable in the past, our gentle approach to uncovering these signals proves how pleasant and helpful they can truly be. Just as your body lets you know when it's time to sleep and when you've rested enough, you can learn to recognize and trust your body signals when it comes to eating.

If you haven't noticed these cues yet, that's okay—you will soon, as you've been reverse engineering your hunger and fullness signals by creating habits and routines that slowly reveal how much food your body truly needs, peeling back the layers one bite at a time.

In the journey toward food freedom, our relationship with hunger and fullness has deep-rooted spiritual applications. Throughout the Bible—from Eve and Adam in Eden to Jesus Christ in the wilderness, and from the Israelites during the exodus from Egypt to Daniel in Babylon—the need to eat has often served as a divine test of obedience. This connection underscores the spiritual significance of our interactions with food, reminding us that even our eating habits can reflect our faith and responsiveness to God's guidance.

He Feeds Us Just Enough

God designed us with the need to eat as a way to deepen our trust in his provision. As Matthew 6:26 says, "Look at the birds of the air: they neither sow nor reap nor gather into barns, and yet your heavenly Father feeds them. Are you not of more value than they?" This verse reminds us of God's continual care, a concept that even the Israelites struggled to remember despite witnessing miracles such as the parting of the Red Sea.

In Exodus 16, after a month of wandering in the wilderness, the Israelites' hunger caused them to look back on their time in Egypt with a sense of longing, forgetting the fact that it was a land of imprisonment and slavery. This reminds us how easily we can romanticize past experiences, overlooking their painful aspects—a trap I often fell into whenever I was lured back into dieting again. Like me, God's chosen people grumbled, complained, and overly dramatized their situation: "[If only] we had died by the hand of the LORD in the land of Egypt, when we sat by the meat pots and ate bread to the full, for you have brought us out into this wilderness to kill this whole assembly with hunger" (Exod. 16:3).

Although God was displeased with their complaining and lack of faith, he provided exactly what they needed. "Then the LORD said to Moses, 'Behold, I am about to rain bread from heaven for you, and the people shall go out and gather a day's portion every day, that I may test them, whether they will walk in my law or not'" (v. 4). The Israelites were told to gather just enough—no more, no less—as means to reveal their obedience. Some chose to ignore these instructions and stashed away extra portions, likely out of mistrust. By the next morning, the bread they saved was found rotten and crawling with maggots.

Ever felt like that after overeating? Yeah, me too!

The real issue wasn't them saving food; it was how that act revealed their lack of trust in God's goodness as a loving Father. Our Father wants us to have good things, if we are willing to wait.

From "Starving" to "Stuffed"

I don't know about you, but hunger and I had a broken relationship. I was so afraid of being hungry that I'd stuff my purse with snacks or become anxious when mealtime approached and there was no plan to eat. Hunger was uncomfortable, and I dreaded it—for good reason.

Undereating, imbalanced meals, and stress around food choices (aka diets) can make our hunger cues feel unnatural—loud, bossy, and dread-worthy, as blood glucose swings are quite unpleasant. When those glucose levels dip too low, the body responds by releasing cortisol, which can further dysregulate blood glucose levels, intensifying the cycle of hunger and stress.

And so I lived a life of hunger extremes—eating before I was hungry or ignoring my hunger signals only to get sidelined by a ravenous appetite. Therefore, my "stop eating" signal was mysterious as well. If we're "starving," it's easy to blow past comfortable fullness and end up stuffed. On the flip side, if we eat without being physically hungry, it's hard to tell when we've had enough, since the easiest way to gauge fullness is when hunger fades. That's why emotional eating never quenches our appetites.

Two Sides of the Same Coin

In this chapter, you'll focus on *either* eating when you're hungry *or* stopping when you're full. Why just one? Trying to eat when you're hungry *and* stop when you're full, most of the time, is the Olympics of body-directed eating—it takes time and lots of practice. It's far more manageable and productive to hone in on first one and then the other. And I think you'll be pleasantly surprised to find that once you get comfortable with the first, the second starts to fall into place naturally, since these two habits are quite synergistic in nature.

For example:

- If you wait to eat until you're hungry, it will be much easier to stop when you've had enough, as the cessation of hunger is a notable sign of fullness.
- If you wait longer than usual to eat, you might get extra hungry and end up eating more than usual.
- If you stop eating your meal sooner, you'll find that you're hungry again earlier.
- If you eat a bit past fullness, your hunger will come a little later than usual.

All of this means there's no way to mess up: Eat more than you need, and your body will adjust. Undershoot, and you'll eat more later.

Over time, you'll learn how to use these skills to navigate your daily activities. That's how your appetite can work for you outside of all-or-nothing thinking.

Don't Turn This into a Diet

If you've ever tried intuitive eating, where the primary focus is following your body's eating cues, you know how overwhelming and even diet-like that hyperfocus on bodily signals can feel. After

──── A WORD ON MINDFUL EATING ────

Before you learn about this chapter's habits, let's take a moment to revisit our chapter 3 habit, the Mind-Body Scan, and discuss its relevance to mindful eating (and therefore, hunger and fullness). Whether the Mind-Body Scan has become a regular part of your routine or you could use a quick refresher, now's the perfect time to reflect on its value in helping to decode hunger and fullness through mindful eating.

Mindful eating isn't about perfection or adhering to rigid rules; it's about being a little more present and engaged with what you consume than you were before. Rather than striving for the unattainable goal of a slow, undistracted twenty-minute meal every time you eat, focus on slightly enhancing your awareness of the flavors, textures, and temperatures of your food. This approach not only increases your mental satisfaction but can also help you uncover new insights into your dietary preferences, such as discovering that a bagel leaves you feeling overstuffed but oatmeal gives you steady energy, or that whole milk yogurt makes your heart sing while nonfat yogurt leaves you longing for Ben and Jerry's. These insights would remain hidden without tuning out the noise and tuning in to your body. Mindful eating also nurtures emotional well-being by easing stress around food choices and offering a moment of self-care, as you allow yourself the time to sit down and truly enjoy your meal.

As you decide which habit to focus on next, consider how you can bring your attention back to the Mind-Body Scan, this time with a specific focus on mealtimes and tuning in to your body's cues. Observation leads to understanding, and learning how your body communicates is essential to nourishing yourself well.

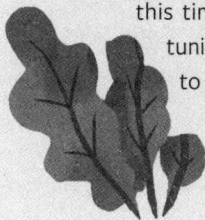

145

years of dieting, trying to unravel what your body needs can feel like decoding a foreign language. You may have even found yourself caught up in perfectionism, obsessing over the ideal timing of hunger and fullness. With the bar set so high, it was easy to stumble and fall into all-or-nothing eating.

Now, with a fresh perspective free from diet mentality, you're prepared to intentionally tune in to what your body needs from a place of self-care. And it can be as easy as revisiting a previous habit with a more attuned focus.

Decoding Hunger and Fullness

You're about to take an important step along the path to food freedom. As you've peeled back the layers of diet baggage, a gentler and more compassionate relationship with your body is beginning to form. You're discovering that it's not just about listening but truly hearing what your body has to say.

This is the connection that will enable you to fuel yourself well, whenever and wherever you go. Whether you're exploring new cuisines on an exotic vacation or scanning casseroles at a church potluck, your body will guide you through your hunger and fullness signals.

As you've started experimenting with portion sizes and balanced meals, you're already laying the foundation for tuning in to your body's natural cues. Consistency in meal timing and composition creates a steady rhythm that makes it easier to identify hunger and fullness.

As you learn more about the habits in this chapter and decide your next step, think of it as Sowing a Seed of Self-Control—growing both your awareness of your body's cues and your willingness to honor them.

Which Should You Choose?

"Should I start with hunger or fullness?" you ask. The answer comes down to two simple questions:

1. Is your eating schedule flexible?
   - **"No, my schedule is not flexible."** If you eat according to a schedule or prioritize family mealtimes, start with Fueling to Fullness. As you become more attuned to your stop signal, you'll begin to reverse engineer your hunger. Correct portion sizes will ensure your body is naturally hungry at your next mealtime.
   - **"Yes, I can pretty much eat when I want."** Move on to question 2.
2. Are you comfortable waiting for hunger?
   - **"Yes, I am ready and excited to experiment with feeling hungry!"** Start with Honing In on Hunger. This habit is ideal for someone with a bit of flexibility in their eating schedule who feels eager to listen to their body's hunger signals.
   - **"Not yet. I'd rather focus on eating less."** Start with Fueling to Fullness. When you tune in to your fullness signals and pay attention to the quantity of food you eat, your hunger signals will naturally start to emerge.

Regardless of what you choose, it's a good idea to review both habits. This will help you make a well-informed decision on where to start, knowing that the end goal is to become fluent in both.

But what if you're still not sure where to start? Or if tuning in to your body's signals feels challenging right now?

Feeling Out of Tune

If your body's cues still feel like a foreign language, it's okay. Long-term sporadic eating habits can make it feel difficult to recognize hunger or fullness signals at first. Try building consistency first. Try to eat within thirty minutes to an hour of waking. Plan meals to occur every three to four hours throughout the day, adjusting earlier if you feel hunger sooner.

This rhythm will encourage your body to rebuild natural hunger and fullness cues over time. If you've been going long stretches without eating, you may find yourself ravenous at meals, making it hard to identify fullness. Regular, balanced meals will gradually help regulate these signals.

Remember, this process takes time—but with a little consistency and a lot of grace, you'll become fluent in your body's unique language before you know it!

Changing Hats

Once again, there's no all-or-nothing in food freedom. Today, you're simply choosing a starting point—one habit for a specific meal or window of time. However, you may find Honing In on Hunger *or* Fueling to Fullness feels more natural at different times. For example, you may cherish family dinners but have some flexibility with breakfast. Begin with whichever "hat" feels right for you, and don't hesitate to switch between them as needed. Over time, you'll find your rhythm, blending both habits to suit your unique needs and preferences.

HABIT 10: HONING IN ON HUNGER

Honing In on Hunger focuses on reconnecting with your body's natural hunger cues. This isn't a white-knuckle approach where you have to rigorously monitor every sensation of appetite or wait in distress until you're allowed to eat. Rather, you're going to gently and purposefully begin to uncover your hunger cues so that you can fall in love with them.

Reframing hunger in a positive light will only help your practice. That gentle pang is a sign your body has exhausted its previous resources and is ready to use some more fuel (rather than store it). Eating when you're hungry also makes it easier to know when you're full, which is an added bonus. But my favorite thing about hunger is how great it makes food taste—hunger is the best seasoning!

Three Ways to Begin

Here are a few options for practicing Honing In on Hunger:

1. **Delay dining, just a bit.** One simple way to begin is to delay your next meal by fifteen minutes. This practice can help you assess if you're truly hungry or if you're opening the refrigerator out of habit. Noticing the physical signs of hunger—like a gentle, pleasant stomach growl—can help you get more comfortable with the feeling. If unsure, a Mind-Body Scan can help you differentiate physical appetite from emotional or habitual eating triggers.

2. **Skip or lighten a snack.** Reducing or skipping the snack prior to your focus meal will let your hunger build more naturally. Notice the tie-in with Fueling to Fullness? Reducing your previous meal's portion size can be a simple way to experience hunger when you'd like to.

3. **Start with the clock.** If you're new to hunger cues, start by using time as a guide. Aim to eat your meals every three or four hours, adjusting earlier if you feel hunger sooner. Around the two or three hour mark, pause and ask yourself, *Am I beginning to feel hungry?* If you don't feel hunger after four hours, consider having a "self-care meal"—a small, balanced meal to gently encourage your body's hunger signals to return. This rhythm helps balance blood sugar while building confidence in recognizing your body's needs.

--- PERSONALIZE YOUR HABIT ---

Now it's time to make this practice your own. Consider how you might begin Honing In on Hunger. Will you wait to eat breakfast until you're hungry? Delay a particular meal each day? Skip an unnecessary snack? Or start with the clock?

Once you've identified your habit, consider what you will do while you are waiting, as a hyperfocus on hunger will only make your habit harder. Then take a moment to jot that plan into your calendar.

Got it? You'll practice this habit for the next week (or longer, if you want to take time to really let it sink in). Be sure to use your free habit tracker and follow along with the included Scripture writing pages to keep your habit and Jesus-first focus front and center.

HABIT 11: FUELING TO FULLNESS

The goal of Fueling to Fullness is to eat enough to satisfy your body's needs—energizing your daily activities without excess that spills over into your "storage."

Fueling to Fullness also means being physically and mentally satiated—able to walk away from the table full, satisfied, energized, and able to move on without thinking about food. Diets have left you longing for more, while overeating made you loathe the thought of another bite. With Fueling to Fullness, you'll seek your middle ground. While you won't nail it right away, each meal will give you more data about what works for you.

Five Tips to Try

Here are a few tips for practicing Fueling to Fullness. Read through them and decide if you'd like one to be your primary habit focus, or simply use them as tools, as needed.

1. **Be a bit more mindful.** As we've discussed, eating mindfully helps boost mental satiety by allowing you to savor the tastes and textures of your meal. Paying attention will also help you recognize your fullness cues, as flavors tend to diminish as your body has enough. Keep in mind it's not

necessary to be mindful and attentive to every single bite. Start small by taking three mindful bites that can serve as anchors or check-in points. You can use these mindful moments independently or in conjunction with the following two tips.

2. **Eat the best bites first.** Instead of saving the best for last, begin your meal with the most appealing bites, whether it's the center of the burger or your favorite part of a salad. This ensures you enjoy the freshest and most flavorful parts of your meal right at the start and reduces your likelihood of overeating at the end when you are already full. Enjoy these bites mindfully to get some extra bang for your buck.

3. **Take a break.** During your meal, take planned breaks either by time (five, seven, and nine minutes in, for example) or as you hit appropriate milestones in your meal, such as one-fourth, half, and three-fourths of the way through. These pauses can help you decide whether to continue eating or if you've had enough.

4. **Eat a bit more slowly.** Slowing down your eating pace can significantly improve your ability to notice when you're full. Consider setting your fork down between bites, using your nondominant hand, or trying a slow-eating app that cues you to chew thoroughly and pause between bites. If you dine with someone who eats more slowly than you do, use their pace as a benchmark to adjust your own plate-to-mouth speed.

5. **Diminish those distractions.** If you watch TV, scroll your phone, or read while you eat, consider working up to undistracted meals by setting aside those distractions for just a few minutes. Then extend that time as your ability to stay present grows. If you're eating with others, bustling conversation can distract too. Use tip 1 and take a few mindful bites.

PERSONALIZE YOUR HABIT

Are you ready to decide how you will practice Fueling to Fullness? Will you simply focus on paying more attention, or will you choose a specific strategy from the list above? Which meal is realistic to begin with? For example, you may be rushing out the door for breakfast but sit down for dinner each night. Start with the easiest option and build upon your success.

Once you know your starting point, consider how you'll remind yourself to implement your habit. If you eat at a specific time, you may set a timer or phone alert to check in with your fullness levels during your meal. A visual cue like a sticky note at your place setting, a fresh bouquet of flowers, or choosing a different seat can serve as a practical reminder. Keep in mind that you'll want to change your reminder from time to time, as it can quickly become too familiar.

Got it? You'll practice this habit for the next week (or longer, if you want to take time to really let it sink in). Be sure to use your free habit tracker and follow along with the included Scripture writing pages to keep your habit and Jesus-first focus front and center.

Hunger and Fullness, in Your Toolbox

"No thanks, I'm not hungry," you say casually, as if you were commenting on the day's weather. You're at a midafternoon training session at church, and naturally, there are cookies. You scan the table for a white chocolate macadamia nut—your favorite—to take home. But today, none of them catch your attention.

It feels good to pass on what you don't want or need. Letting go of expectations and judgments around your eating choices and appetite is one of the best things you could do. After all, there are days when you feel unexpectedly hungry and meals where you get full faster than expected. Being open to what your body needs allows you to fuel yourself well so that you can be fully satisfied.

Of course, no one is perfect. There are also times when you choose to eat even when you're not hungry, like when your child bakes something special for you, or times when you eat a bit more than you wanted because you are engrossed in conversation at the table.

But because there is no dietary tightrope to walk, each meal is just a meal and another opportunity to honor your God-given bodily signals.

Hunger and fullness are becoming your allies, not your enemies.

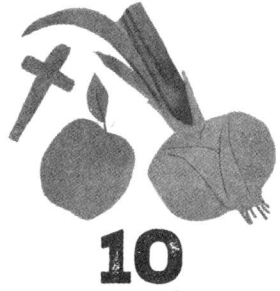

10

HOME BASE HABITS

Let your eyes look directly forward, and your gaze be straight before you. Ponder the path of your feet; then all your ways will be sure.

Proverbs 4:25–26

I was in a groove. Do you know that moment—when all your hard work begins to pay off? Maybe it was when your piano playing started to sound like music or when you had the potential to beat a friend at pickleball. For me, it was my fitness journey.

After years of studying habit change and working as a personal trainer and nutrition coach, I felt like everything was starting to click. I was planning and prepping my meals like a pro, hitting the gym ultra-consistently, and even teaching bootcamp classes.

Then a couple of minor disruptions threw everything off-balance. I injured my knee, and my husband embarked on an elimination diet to manage his rheumatoid arthritis. These seemed like small glitches, but they disrupted my well-laid plans as surely as removing a leg from a chair would topple it.

Perhaps you've experienced something similar—you were carefully following your food plan until vacation left a healthy eating vacancy in its wake, or you were in a great exercise groove until sickness sidelined you and you never found your way back.

That's the nature of all-or-nothing thinking: It's working or it's not. And while we tackled this detrimental mindset in chapter 2, it takes time for those old thinking patterns to dissipate. Even with the progress you've made, traces of all-or-nothing thinking might still linger in your perspective of what makes your habits "successful." And that's okay; I experience this, too, working diligently to acquire routines that feel great, only to start believing that *they* are the secret to my success.

How easy it is to focus on the physical rather than the spiritual.

As you may have noticed, our God does not fit in any boxes, including our expectations or our calendars. If our habits are to be fruitful, they will also need to be elastic to our callings, able to cope with disruptions, and have enough memory to bounce back to what works. That elasticity happens with consistency.

In this chapter, you're going to learn how to identify the habits that offer you the most benefit with the greatest ease. This will allow you to be better prepared for all circumstances. Then, in the next chapter, you'll catch the vision of what lifelong food freedom looks like. These two chapters will equip you with the tools you need to keep moving forward, with your eyes on the prize, no matter what life throws your way.

The Purpose of Your Transformation

You have dreams, goals, and a unique calling that only you can fulfill. At times, it may have felt like your battle with food was a barrier holding you back, hindering your progress. Yet, in God's hands, these struggles become the very tools he uses to refine and prepare you for what's ahead.

God's grace is the foundation of any lasting transformation. By embracing our need for the Savior, we acknowledge that his strength, mercy, and "new morning" fresh starts are gifts we need daily. This truth frees us from the grip of perfectionism and reminds us that God loves us as we are. He also calls us to live fruitful lives as we step into the plans he has for us. He wants to use us for his kingdom purposes and to fulfill the dreams he's placed within our hearts. When we pursue his purposes, including our habits, we can't help but be fruitful.

This understanding helps us recognize that forming our habits starts with seeking God first. As Matthew 6:33 reminds us, when we seek his kingdom and righteousness, all our other needs will be met. Trusting that Christ has already paid the price for our freedom (John 8:36) liberates us from the burden of striving for change on our own. God is the ultimate source of our success, empowering us to release the weight of self-effort and rely on his strength and provision instead.

Most importantly, the ultimate goal of our transformation is to bring glory to God. Why? Because when he is glorified, others are drawn to him.

Too often, I've allowed my food and fitness routines to hold me back from being fully available. Can you relate? On this journey to food freedom, let's commit to staying flexible, allowing our habits to adapt to new seasons and opportunities for service. One practical way to keep this mindset is by developing Home Base Habits—doable, sustainable practices that ground us no matter our life stage or circumstance. These habits allow us to flow with God's plan rather than being rigidly bound to the demands of diet guidelines or even our own habit ideals.

Even on a Hard Day

What if your habits weren't just something you *do* but a reflection of *who you are*? We've talked about how habits are the things we do most of the time, but what if they became so ingrained that they carried you through, even on the difficult days?

Let's say the day's chaos is in full swing—your inbox is flooded with urgent emails, the kids are arguing, and the dog just knocked over a potted plant. Yet in the middle of it all, you find yourself washing greens and prepping a simple salad for lunch. Not because you have to or because you think you should, but because you just *do*.

Or maybe a loved one needs your help, so you end up missing your workout and dinner prep. The only option left is to grab take-out on your way home. But that's okay—instead of overindulging, you marry your wants with wisdom and leave a couple of bites on your plate. Not because you have to or because you feel like you should, but because it feels right . . . and you just *do*.

These are your Home Base Habits.

Your Path to Home Base Habits

Home Base Habits are foundational practices that are familiar, effective, and easy to lean on when life gets messy. They provide maximum benefit without requiring much effort to maintain. With practice, they will run nearly on autopilot, keeping you grounded and aligned with your goals even during challenging times, when you might have given up in the past.

While they'll remain fairly consistent, you may adjust them as you grow and change. Most of the time, you'll be adding new habits to your routine, which we'll explore in the next chapter. However, there will also be moments when it's best to scale back to your Home Base Habits, such as these:

Your time and energy are limited. Whether your limits are due to illness, caregiving, or life transitions like moving or job changes, these habits will help you maintain stability, preserve your emotional reserves, and ensure self-care when you need it most.

You need a mental break. You've been working diligently on your healthy habits, and sometimes you need a pause. When you want a breather without backsliding, taking a week to reset with your Home Base Habits can help you regain focus and feel refreshed.

You're out of your regular routine. Vacations, holidays, or unexpected changes can throw off your schedule. Instead of letting everything slide, you can rely on these simple, doable habits to keep things steady.

You moved too fast. If you've been overzealous in adding new habits and feel overwhelmed, scaling back to your Home Base Habits will help you regain consistency. From there, you can slowly and sustainably add other habits back in, as you're ready.

You don't have to fear disruptions, distractions, or drudgery, as you're always free to pare back to your foundational habits whenever you want or need to.

Discovering Your Home Base Habits

Before we work to uncover your Home Base Habits, let's take a moment to reflect on your existing habits from this journey and explore each as a potential Home Base Habit. This will serve both as a refresher and an opportunity to weigh the effectiveness and ease of each one for you. (As some chapters included two habits to choose from, you may not have completed every single one.)

Fully Nourished Habit Recap

Habit 1: Grow in Gratitude

Establishing an intentional gratitude practice helps train your heart and mind to recognize and focus on the goodness of God and the blessings he's given you. This practice creates a more peaceful and joyful internal environment, allowing you to navigate life's challenges with greater calm and resilience, reducing the urge to emotionally eat.

Habit 2: Sowing Seeds of Self-Control

This habit's flexibility makes it an ideal travel companion or a primary focus, as it embodies the heart of *Fully Nourished*. Though what we can offer the Lord may seem small, when given in faith, with our whole heart, he can grow it into more than we ask, imagine, or think. Sowing Seeds of Self-Control can adapt to any season of life—honing in on how you eat or responding to another area the Lord is nudging you to grow in.

Habit 3: Mind-Body Scan

Harness the power of a pause. Recall the difference in your meals when you take a moment to tune in to your fullness levels or how much lighter your emotions feel when you acknowledge them before they build up. By simply giving yourself the gift of a pause, you create space to hear the quiet nudges of your body, the subtle calls for self-care, and the still, small voice of the Holy Spirit.

Habit 4: Simply Plan Ahead

As we've discovered, obsessing over what we eat is draining, but giving no thought to our meals isn't helpful either. Taking some time to plan your meals—whether that's a weekly meal plan, daily eats, or anything in between—positions you to nourish yourself well. Simply Plan Ahead can act as an umbrella, covering other practices such as your Food Quality or Balancing Out Your Plate habit. A little forethought goes a long way.

Habit 5: Grow Fruitful Habits

Much like Sowing Seeds of Self-Control, the practice of working to Grow Fruitful Habits adapts to your needs and preferences. The only requirement is that your habit should serve and support you well—be it a food freedom habit or one unique to you.

Habit 6: Fruit-Filled Journaling

The battle for our hearts begins in our minds, as our self-talk and beliefs shape the quality and direction of our lives. Mind-renewal requires intention, and by taking just a few minutes each day to examine your thoughts, you can capture runaway thoughts and replace them with biblical truth (2 Cor. 10:5) rather than allowing unchecked mental scripts to steer you off course.

Habits 7 and 8: Food Quality or Food Quantity

These two habits were introduced in the same chapter, so you could choose the focus that felt most comfortable and productive for you. I use both of these as my Home Base Habits, utilizing one or both as the situation calls. Real food fuels me best, so I prioritize Food Quality when I can. However, there are times when my choices are limited, so keeping tabs on Food Quantity is an excellent strategy. It's up to you if one or both make your roster.

Habit 9: Balance Out Your Plate

As you lay down your diet baggage, nutrition knowledge becomes a valuable tool rather than a burdensome have-to. In the past, you may have felt rebellious toward rigid eating guidelines, resisting off-limits foods only to cave in with disappointment later. But now it's clear that some of that dissatisfaction came from imbalanced meals—plates missing a good mix of macronutrients. If you've felt significantly better after adjusting your plate proportions, this could be a Home Base Habit for you.

Habits 10 and 11: Honing In on Hunger or Fueling to Fullness

This chapter empowered you to choose between Honing In on Hunger or Fueling to Fullness, allowing you to find rest in a simplified and focused practice. You've learned that these two signals flex and flow in response to each other, encouraging you to let go of perfectionism and build trust in your body. While mastering these skills takes time, the process of listening to your body's cues is a powerful proficiency worth nurturing.

As you can see, these habits cover a lot of ground! But as always, on your journey to food freedom, you're not boxed in to any set of rules. The quiz below will give you the chance to reflect on these habits while also adding your own ideas. In the end, you'll develop a personalized set of Home Base Habits you feel confident committing to. Then, in the next chapter, you'll learn how to customize your habit practice further, building upon your foundation like a pro.

Assessing Your Home Base Habits

Who doesn't love a good quiz? Let's pinpoint which habits serve you well. Grab two different colored pens—one for Effectiveness and one for Ease. Then follow the instructions below to rate each habit.

Use your **Effectiveness** color to circle the number that reflects how fruitful each habit has been and how it supports your goals and well-being.

Use your **Ease** color to circle the number that shows how doable and sustainable that habit has felt in your daily life.

By visually assessing your habits in this way, you'll quickly identify which ones are both beneficial and manageable.

0 = NOT effective and NOT easy
10 = Effective AND easy

Grow in Gratitude	0-1-2-3-4-5-6-7-8-9-10
Sowing Seeds of Self-Control	0-1-2-3-4-5-6-7-8-9-10
Mind-Body Scan	0-1-2-3-4-5-6-7-8-9-10
Simply Plan Ahead	0-1-2-3-4-5-6-7-8-9-10
Grow Fruitful Habits	0-1-2-3-4-5-6-7-8-9-10

Fruit-Filled Journaling	0-1-2-3-4-5-6-7-8-9-10
Food Quality Path	0-1-2-3-4-5-6-7-8-9-10
Food Quantity Path	0-1-2-3-4-5-6-7-8-9-10
Balance Out Your Plate	0-1-2-3-4-5-6-7-8-9-10
Honing In on Hunger	0-1-2-3-4-5-6-7-8-9-10
Fueling to Fullness	0-1-2-3-4-5-6-7-8-9-10

Now that you've rated your habits, cast your net a bit wider to consider other habits that you may find beneficial. Some examples are:

Bible study

prayer

drinking water

leaving three bites on your plate

regular movement or exercise

bedtime/sleep schedules

self-care practices (e.g., afternoon nap or weekly massage)

eating slowly

pausing during meals

undistracted dining

Write them in and assess them with your two colors below:

_____	0-1-2-3-4-5-6-7-8-9-10
_____	0-1-2-3-4-5-6-7-8-9-10
_____	0-1-2-3-4-5-6-7-8-9-10
_____	0-1-2-3-4-5-6-7-8-9-10
_____	0-1-2-3-4-5-6-7-8-9-10

You may want to pause here and take a moment to pray over your quiz. Is something missing? Does one of your ratings feel slightly off? While there's no need to overanalyze, sitting with this assessment may allow your assumptions and unrealistic expectations to soften and yield to the truth.

⬛⬛⬛⬛⬛

Now, looking over your lists, which habits won in effectiveness *and* ease? Jot the top three to five down in your journal. Next to each one, describe what it would look like day-to-day, why it is helpful, and how you will cue yourself to complete it. For example, you may choose Grow in Gratitude. This habit helps you maintain a positive outlook and reduce internal tension in just a few minutes. It's also tied in to your morning Bible time, making it so ingrained that you hardly have to think about doing it now.

Maybe you pick Fueling to Fullness. If you have an active social life through church or other community involvement, perhaps you love how this habit helps you stay mindful of your portions, no matter what food is being served. The best part? You can keep it simple by checking in with yourself halfway through your meal and giving a little extra attention as you approach the three-quarters mark, helping you reach comfortable fullness without feeling restricted.

Or maybe you choose to Balance Out Your Plate through having a whole-food breakfast. This meal is simple to preplan on the weekends when you're reviewing your calendar, and you've noticed that starting your day with a quality breakfast sets you up for success. It keeps your energy steady and your cravings at bay, helping you sail smoothly from breakfast right to lunch.

Are you beginning to see which habits are the most fruitful and easiest for you? Let me remind you once more: While you want to be thoughtful in this process, there's absolutely no need for perfection. Your Home Base Habits aren't set in stone; they can and likely will evolve as your life and needs change.

Simply do your best, pick the habits that feel right for now, and start solidifying your foundation!

Pick Your Home Base Habits

The top three habits you've selected are your Home Base Habits. I encourage you to practice them with intention and curiosity over the next couple of weeks. Notice how they fit into your day and how they make you feel. These habits are meant to provide a strong foundation you can return to when life gets hectic or when you need to recalibrate. They're also the routines you'll build upon as you continue to grow and evolve through your food freedom journey.

The key to Home Base Habits is consistency. You're looking for them to become so ingrained in your routine that they happen almost automatically, even on your most challenging days. Of course, developing habits like these takes practice, and that's exactly the gift you're giving yourself right now.

Be sure to use your free habit tracker and follow along with the included Scripture writing pages to keep your habits and Jesus-first focus front and center.

When Habits Become Second Nature

We didn't expect it. We never really do, do we?

Life's unexpected turns seem to pop up out of nowhere. But Jesus told us not to worry about tomorrow because today has enough trouble of its own (Matt. 6:34). And yes, we'll see our fair share of tribulation.

In the past, when the stress hit, like that time your washer flooded the house *and* you ended up with two flat tires, everything healthy in your life would derail. But today, something feels different.

Sure, you'd rather be lounging on a beach in Maui, but just because you locked your keys in the car on the same day you twisted your ankle while walking the dog doesn't mean your self-care goes out the window.

Not anymore.

You still managed to get in your Fruit-Filled Journaling (mostly while icing your ankle), left a few bites of your taco salad when you felt satisfied, and refilled your water bottle three times.

The old you would have let these challenges throw you off course, but no longer. Today, you're operating on well-ingrained habits that don't require the perfect day to stay in motion. You don't need to wait for tomorrow to start fresh, although you're definitely looking forward to it.

This was just another day of living like the new you.

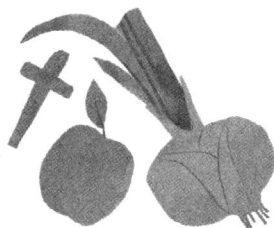

11

HOW TO STAY FREE

So Jesus said to the Jews who had believed him, "If you abide in my word, you are truly my disciples, and you will know the truth, and the truth will set you free."

John 8:31–32

I sat down at my kitchen table, pen in hand, ready to work through the thoughts swirling in my mind. Yes, I know a paper journal is old school, but I needed the time to process as I wrote. Seeing my ruminations laid out in front of me gave me the space I needed to reflect.

Have you noticed that too? It's like organizing a cluttered drawer—overwhelming at first, but once you empty its contents, sorting it out becomes much easier.

I had spent the last two weeks trying to stop eating after dinner, but it just wasn't happening, and frustration was creeping in. *Why is this so hard?*

I thought avoiding a nighttime snack was important to me. I didn't like going to bed too full, and I knew I didn't need the extra calories, yet I couldn't seem to stop this habit. *What's my problem?*

I set my pen down, rested my head in my hands, and took a moment to pause. It was clear this self-interrogation was only making me more defensive, so I decided to step back. I breathed deeply, exhaling my irritation, then prayed a quick prayer for wisdom, put on my coach's hat, and became a gentle but curious observer of myself.

What is my favorite part about my nighttime snack? I asked myself calmly. *And if I don't eat it, what am I afraid will happen?*

Isn't it interesting how things change when we stop judging ourselves and start listening? I realized I was more attached to that evening snack—usually yogurt with berries—than I'd thought. The truth was, I didn't actually want to give it up. I was only trying because I felt like I *should*. And that sense of obligation was making me cling to "my treat" even tighter.

Clearly, my approach wasn't working. If my real goal was to go to bed feeling comfortable and to be more mindful of my food quantity, then maybe there was another way to get there. With this new mindset, I found a better solution: Instead of trying to eliminate my after-dinner eating, I decided to tune in more carefully to my fullness levels at dinner, leaving room for the snack *if* I truly wanted it.

That moment affirmed for me that food freedom isn't about forcing ourselves to follow "shoulds" or rigid rules; it's about partnering with the Lord to discover what truly works. That day, I chose to enjoy my evening snack without any guilt. And you know what's interesting? Now I only snack after dinner a couple of times a week, and I never go to bed feeling too full.

Food freedom is not a passive process, but don't confuse activity with progress. Keep in mind: The busyness of diets got you nowhere. And I think you'll discover that, oftentimes, the most productive work is slowing down, praying, and asking the right questions. Change rarely happens without resistance. So instead of pushing through that resistance, what if you approached it with curiosity?

Just as God's grace leads us in our journey of faith, he also guides us in these everyday struggles. After all, hard things are hard until they become easy—gentleness is the key to unlocking opposition.

In the same way it takes time for new habits to form, it takes time for old habits to fade away.

Avoiding the Drift

Let's take a moment to consider your *Fully Nourished* habits. When you first started your Grow in Gratitude habit, it likely took extra effort to plan and follow through with your intention. Some days you nailed it, and other days it slipped your mind.

But over time, with practice and consistency, writing that gratitude list got easier. Perhaps now it's a natural part of your day, something you barely think about anymore.

But even if that habit is still finding its footing, you've likely seen how other habits, once difficult, can eventually become so ingrained that you practically do them on autopilot. And that's the ultimate goal for any habit: Find a meaningful aim that aligns with your goals and values (one that is doable, sustainable, appealing, and effective), practice it with intention until it becomes easy enough to do *most days* (without a lot of effort), then move on to the next one.

But as you and I both know, old habits—the ones you're trying to leave behind, especially those ingrained over the years—don't require much effort either. And they can subtly pull you off course if you're not paying attention. Like floating in the ocean, you don't realize you've drifted until you look up and see your towel is now a tiny dot on the shore. Habits work the same way; without focus, we can unknowingly drift back to old patterns.

That's how habits are designed to work. It doesn't mean you're broken, and you're not doing anything wrong. You just need a strategy to manage the drift. You can prevent it through intentional reflection and recalibration. In this chapter, you'll discover how to stay aligned with your habits and routines using the simple, effective strategies I've used to coach women for over a decade. You'll walk away feeling empowered, equipped for the next step, and confident in your ability to keep moving forward.

Stay Free by Checking In

As you've learned by now, one of the greatest gifts you can give yourself is *time*—time to learn, time to grow, and time to pause. Like many of us, I used to rush through life, constantly pushing myself to be "productive" in an attempt to prove my worth and value. This led to burnout, exhaustion, and ultimately neglecting what mattered most to me.

Now, you and I are learning a new truth: Our worth is secure in Christ. We don't need to perform or achieve to prove our value. Our highest calling is to abide in him, which enables us to listen to his guidance in every area of life, including our habits.

A Fully Nourished Check-In will equip you to do just that. As you reflect on how your habits are going—pausing to pray and tune in to God's direction—you'll gain clarity on your next steps. You'll avoid drifting off course and investing your precious time in habits that no longer serve you. You'll also ensure that the habits you practice bring you closer to both your goals and your calling, thereby strengthening your journey to freedom.

This check-in is a simple yet powerful way to reflect on your progress and plan for the days ahead. It includes answering a series of questions, either weekly or biweekly, based on your needs. At first, it will take you about thirty minutes, but as you get familiar with the process, you'll likely complete it in fifteen minutes or less.

During this focused time, you'll review your habits, recognize what's working, make necessary adjustments, and set your next steps. It's an opportunity to troubleshoot, prepare, and refocus—all in one quick session. This check-in will be one of the best investments you'll make in your journey to food freedom. You may even enjoy it so much that you turn it into a personal ritual—perhaps grabbing a coffee, sitting in a quiet spot, and prayerfully reviewing not just your habits but your entire week ahead.

Below are the nine questions you'll review during your check-in time. You can jot them down in a journal or download the free check-in sheet provided with this book.

——— MY FULLY NOURISHED CHECK-IN ———

1. What habit(s) have I been practicing?
Take note of the habit(s) you've focused on since your last check-in. Be specific; this will help when you look back over your progress and analyze what's working—and what's not. Remember, it's all useful data!

2. Share a WIN!
No matter what kind of week you've had, there's always something positive to highlight. This practice trains your eyes to see the good and helps cultivate a heart of gratitude.

3. What fruit did this habit bear? What would I like to keep doing?
Consider the results of your habit. Did it produce positive fruit such as peace, joy, or better health? By recognizing the benefits, you'll be more motivated to continue doing what's working.

4. What would I like to do differently?
There's always room for learning. Reflect on what didn't work and use it as a stepping stone for growth. Mistakes are not setbacks; they're opportunities to improve.

5. What habit(s) would I like to practice?
Choose what you'll focus on until your next check-in. Lean on your Home Base Habits or consider introducing a new one. If you're unsure, revisit your previous check-in or review all eleven Fully Nourished habits and your Fruitful Habits list. Remember, your habit does not need to be food-focused. Other activities that enrich or simplify your life will benefit your relationship with food!

6. On a scale of 1–10, how confident am I that I can nail this habit?
(*If less than an 8, adjust until you're confident.*)
Your goal is to choose a habit that's doable, sustainable, appealing, and effective. Make adjustments to set yourself up for success!

7. What challenges do I foresee?

What factors could make your habit more difficult? Are there any scheduling challenges you'll want to be aware of? Are there busy days when you'll need to simplify your meals or pack a snack? Do you see any room for self-care? A little preparation goes a long way in avoiding unnecessary stress. Remember, you're aiming for progress, not perfection: Start easy, do your best, and learn from both your successes and setbacks.

8. How will I address those challenges?

You don't need a complex plan, just one or two simple actions. Set a reminder on your phone, adjust your schedule, or pencil in some self-care to refresh yourself when you'll need it most.

9. Choose a Bible verse for the upcoming week(s).

Let Scripture guide and encourage you as you practice your habit. Select a verse to be your plumb line as you move forward.

Not sure what to pick? A quick online search for Bible verses about the challenge mentioned in the last question (managing stress, motivation, relationships, etc.) can help you find a solid place to stand.

These simple but powerful questions can provide valuable insight into your habits, helping you assess their effectiveness and plan for what's next.

Frequently Asked Questions

Now, I bet you've got some questions! Below, you'll find a list of those I hear often. Skim the sections and read those that resonate with you, or review them all for added clarity. Then we'll get your first check-in scheduled, and I'll leave you with some final words of encouragement.

How Often Should I Check In?

Ideally, you'll want to check in weekly or biweekly. But how do you decide which frequency works best for you? Let's break it down.

Weekly check-ins: If you opt to check in weekly, you'll have the benefit of keeping your habits at the forefront of your mind. This frequency helps you tackle challenges as they arise in real time and prevents you from drifting too far from your goals. However, a week is not long enough to fully assess whether a new habit is effective (unless it's clearly *not* working). So, with weekly check-ins, be prepared to practice patience and give your habits time to develop. If you're in a season of focusing primarily on Home Base Habits, a weekly check-in may feel too often.

Biweekly check-ins: If you check in every two weeks, you'll have more time to evaluate how a habit is working. This schedule allows you to notice patterns, brainstorm adjustments based on real experiences, and make thoughtful decisions. However, if you need to adjust a habit midstream, waiting two weeks might delay important changes.

For most people, I recommend starting with weekly check-ins. Once you're comfortable with the process and feel that your habits are solidifying, you can move to biweekly check-ins.

Do I Need to Add Any Other Steps to My Journey?

Great question! If you're anything like me and have a history of jumping from one diet plan to the next, you might find yourself constantly asking, "What's next?" It's completely normal; years of dieting condition us to believe that progress always requires something new or more extreme. But here's the liberating truth:

the concepts in *Fully Nourished* can absolutely be enough to help you reach your goals!

Remember how we talked in chapter 7 about the fact that diets can only do two things, adjust your food quantity or your food quality? You're either improving what you eat or changing how much you consume. That is just one of the small steps you've learned during this journey to food freedom. Now, using what you've already learned, imagine a slow, sustainable approach where you continually fine-tune these areas. Over time, this steady progress not only helps you meet your goals but also ensures you can maintain those changes long-term.

By also staying mindful of your hunger and fullness signals and choosing Fruitful Habits that align with your values, you're setting yourself up for lasting change. This approach is far more effective and fulfilling than any trendy diet plan because it's built on what truly works for *you*.

Diet plans tend to push you too far, too fast, often prescribing changes that aren't even necessary for you to reach your goals. For example, jumping onto a low-carb diet might restrict you more than needed, leading to unnecessary limitations. But if you simply tweak your carbohydrate portions—adjusting just enough to maximize both satiety and energy—you can see results without any drastic measures.

In short, you don't need to add anything more unless it aligns with your unique goals and journey. Becoming fully nourished is about discovering what truly works for you, not what diets prescribe! However, if you find yourself struggling to implement your habits or need extra guidance, a counselor or registered dietitian can help guide you into your next steps.

How Will I Know If I've Reached My Goals?

When weight loss is the primary goal, the end point seems crystal clear: Reach a certain number on the scale, and you're done. But much like a mirage, that goal often moves further away, always just out of reach. So, when your focus shifts to food freedom, how will you know when you've arrived? And what if you still have health and weight loss goals? Can both coexist?

Food freedom is measured by a progression of peace. In my experience recovering from binge eating and overeating, I didn't wake up one day and realize I had "arrived." Instead, my progress was marked by less frequent binges that were also less intense and had a quicker recovery. The journey was not about crossing a line from struggle to freedom but a gradual rise to more ease and joy around food.

When it comes to weight loss, a primary focus on numbers will distract you from finding long-term, sustainable habits that fit your life—the ones that will get you to your happy place and keep you there. As you implement these habits, many will naturally become part of your routine because they're easy, enjoyable, and even second nature. Over time, you'll arrive at a crossroads where your goals and sustainability align: You'll feel satisfied with your current habits, and the idea of making further changes seems undesirable or disruptive to your food freedom.

For example, imagine you're feeling happy in your own skin— partially because you've lost some weight, but more because your body image has transformed. You've learned to appreciate your body as a gift from the Lord and you're eating healthier than ever, finding joy in trying new recipes while still making space for family pizza nights and a daily sweet treat. Sure, you could tighten up your portion sizes or cut back on some indulgences, but that feels too restrictive and not worth sacrificing your food peace over.

This is when you know you've found your stopping point: To go further would actually pull you back into an unhealthy relationship with food.

What If My Habit Isn't Working?

When a habit becomes a struggle or never gains traction, it can be frustrating. But, as we've discovered, this is valuable data—a chance to reflect, reassess, and adjust so you can keep progressing.

Often, if a habit isn't working, it comes down to one of four main reasons:

1. **You don't really want to do this habit.** Sometimes we choose habits based on what we *think* we should do or because they worked for us in the past. But if you're struggling to stay consistent, it might be because this habit doesn't align with your current needs. Take a step back from assumptions and ask yourself, *What do I genuinely want or need in this season?* Then revisit chapter 4, "Uncover the Goals That Motivate You," to reconnect with what truly matters to you.

2. **Your habit is too big or too small.** If your habit feels overwhelming, it's possible you fell into some unrealistic expectations about what your life can handle right now. Scale it back until you're at least an 8 out of 10 confident you can achieve what you've set out to do. On the flip side, if your habit feels uninspiring or too easy, you may have pulled back too far. Amp it up slightly to reignite your motivation. The key is finding a habit that feels doable but still pushes you toward growth without becoming overwhelming.

3. **You've slipped back into the diet mindset.** Feeling discouraged, stuck in all-or-nothing thinking, or shaming yourself for missing the mark? Those old dieting demands may have crept back in. Remember, food freedom isn't about being perfect—it's about grace and steady progress. If the diet mindset is slipping back in, revisit chapter 2, "Reject the Diet Mentality," for a reminder about the awesome power and necessity of grace.

4. **The root cause is something deeper.** Sometimes fumbles have nothing to do with the habit. Stress, relationship issues, or even a lack of joy in your life can be the underlying

factors. Instead of focusing solely on the habit, take a moment to ask yourself what's really going on. By addressing your deeper needs—whether that's rest, emotional care, or spiritual support—you'll uncover a habit focus that will yield more transformative results.

When your habit isn't working, don't be discouraged! Use this as a time to assess, adjust, and lean in to God's grace as you continue to move forward. Just like with any journey, there will be bumps along the way, but with a little reflection and recalibration, you'll keep progressing toward food freedom.

How Will I Know If I'm Ready for a New Habit?

When you're practicing your habit, it's essential to check in regularly to evaluate its effectiveness and whether or not you're ready to take on something new. Here's how to know if you're ready for a new habit:

1. **You're consistent and comfortable.** If your current habit feels manageable, and you're practicing it regularly without much effort or resistance, it might be time to add on. Ask yourself, *Does this habit feel almost automatic now? Do I feel confident with it most days?*
2. **The habit feels sustainable.** Does this habit feel like something you can do long-term? If it's doable, and you're seeing positive results (even small ones), this may be a sign you're ready for the next step.
3. **You've learned from your experience.** Sometimes, even when a habit isn't a great fit, the lessons you've learned from it can guide your next steps. Reflect on how you've grown through this practice. Have you gained insight into what works for you and what doesn't? If yes, then you're prepared to either continue refining this habit or take on a new one that better suits your current needs.

If you feel good about where you're at but aren't sure about moving forward, take some time to pray and listen for direction. You'll know you're ready for the next habit when you feel peace about moving ahead and confidence that your current habit is stable enough to support the new one.

Help, I'm Not Losing Weight! What Do I Do?

If you're not seeing the weight loss progress you expected, it's important to start by reviewing your current habit lineup. Inconsistent habits often lead us to jump to conclusions about what's working or not. For example, you may nail your habits during the week but not the weekend. To assume that your habits won't lead to weight loss would be based on inaccurate data.

Look for habits you can be consistent with first.

Before we dive into practical tips, let's remember that while it's okay to desire weight loss, we never want to make losing weight our primary goal, as we'll never find contentment on the scale. If you're struggling with body image, revisit chapter 3, "Align Your Body Image with God's Word."

Now, here are six key areas to assess if your weight loss has stalled. Maybe you'll find your next habit below!

1. **Your perceptions of hunger and fullness are off.** Are you accurately assessing hunger and fullness? Sometimes our perceptions are skewed from years of dieting, leading us to fear hunger—eating at the first shadow of a hunger pang or eating more than we need to avoid feeling hungry later. Experiment with waiting fifteen more minutes before eating to distinguish true hunger from a craving, or try leaving a few bites on your plate. Small, doable tweaks like this, practiced consistently, can lead to steady progress as you uncover how much food your body really needs to thrive.

2. **You could use a quality upgrade.** If your body signals
   are on track but the scale isn't budging, take a moment to
   evaluate your food quality. Calorie for calorie, processed
   foods tend to be less satisfying than their whole-food coun-
   terparts. Play around with upgrading your food quality or
   revisit chapter 8, "Nutrition Made Simple," for ways to
   tweak your plate and see how your satiety signals respond.

3. **You're dehydrated.** Dehydration can mimic hunger, which
   can lead to unnecessary snacking. Ideally, aim to drink
   half your body weight in ounces of water daily (e.g., if
   you weigh 150 pounds, aim for 75 ounces). If your current
   water intake is low, gradually increase it over the course of
   a couple of weeks to give your system time to adjust. Staying hydrated not only helps manage cravings but also supports digestion, helps maintain optimal body function, and
   boosts your energy levels.

4. **You're tired.** Sleep is often overlooked but has a profound
   impact on weight loss. Without adequate rest, your body
   struggles to regulate hunger hormones like ghrelin and
   leptin, leading to increased cravings. It also impairs your
   ability to focus on healthy habits, pushing you to seek
   quick energy boosts from sugar, processed carbs, and caf-
   feine. If you're getting less than seven hours of sleep a
   night, focus on improving your sleep quantity or quality.
   Establish a bedtime routine by going to bed at the same
   time, reducing screen time before sleep, and keeping your
   bedroom dark, cool, and quiet. Even if sleep doesn't come
   easily, prioritizing rest can restore your energy and help
   your body reset.

5. **You're stressed.** Stress can derail even our best efforts.
   When your body is in a constant state of stress, digestion
   slows and cravings for comfort foods (usually high in sugar
   or fat) intensify. Chronic stress can also lead to emotional

eating, which often interferes with weight loss goals. A habit that focuses on stress management may be just what you need. Practice Fruit-Filled Journaling and find moments of peace in your day by engaging in activities that replenish you, such as taking walks, practicing gratitude, or spending quiet time in God's Word.

6. **Your mindset isn't helping.** Weight loss isn't always immediate, and it's essential to approach it with patience and grace, as negative self-talk can sabotage your efforts. Thoughts like *I deserve this treat* or *I'll never lose weight* can keep you stuck in destructive patterns. Don't fight your negative thoughts; instead, counter them with the truth. Revisit chapter 6, "Let Go of What Holds You Back," reading it through the lens of your current self-talk struggles.

Get Started with Your First Fully Nourished Check-In

Now it's time to shift focus to your check-ins so that you can get your first one on the calendar! Your questions are often answered through prayer and reflection—two things facilitated by your Fully Nourished Check-Ins. Are you ready? Let's go!

Step 1: Schedule your first check-in.

Is there a time in the next week when you can set aside thirty minutes to complete your initial check-in? Why thirty minutes? You'll want to take your time to get the most out of these nine questions. With practice, you'll likely complete them more quickly.

Step 2: Set a recurring appointment with yourself.

Looking over the next few months, is there a day and time you feel you could pretty consistently complete your check-in? Ideally, look for a time that is anchored to another habit, such as planning your upcoming week or waiting while your kiddos are at soccer practice.

These appointments with yourself will be the habit you can hang your food freedom on, as you prayerfully seek your next steps, never veering too far from your intention.

As you move forward with the tools and insights you've gained, remember that food freedom is an ongoing journey, not a one-time achievement. It's a walk of progress, grace, and constant growth. And while the road may not always be smooth, you have everything you need to stay on the path toward peace, joy, and true freedom in Christ.

YOU: FREE

How I wish we could sit together over a cup of coffee and catch up on your journey. You'd tell me about how your struggles with food began—maybe after a hurtful comment in middle school, or perhaps following the birth of your first child. I'd see the lingering pain in your eyes from years of battling food, feeling like freedom was out of reach and wondering if you were ever truly "enough."

But as you share more of your story, we'd both begin to notice the unmistakable threads of Jesus woven throughout. His divine direction has been with you all along, never allowing you to settle for anything less than the freedom his blood purchased for you. Perhaps there would be a few tears—not of regret, but of release. The sadness and guilt that once weighed you down so heavily would be gently washed away, replaced by the peace that surpasses understanding, ushering in a deep sense of hope.

We'd talk about your journey through *Fully Nourished*. You'd share how you've started to see yourself through God's eyes—how you've learned to invite him into every part of your process, and how food no longer holds the same power over you. You'd reflect on the freedom you've found from the endless cycle of guilt and shame. You've grown in gratitude and grace, embracing the truth that progress, not perfection, is the goal.

Of course, we both know there's still room for growth—there always will be until we meet Jesus face-to-face. But you'd share how, even in your ongoing struggles, you're learning to lean on your Savior more and more. I'd remind you that even your toughest days can be victorious if they point you back to him.

Every step you've taken, every pause for reflection, has brought you closer to peace and freedom in your relationship with food.

Yes, the road ahead will have highs and lows—challenges, doubts, and moments when old habits try to sneak back in. But you're not the same person who started this journey. You're equipped with tools rooted in truth, empowered by grace, and guided by the wisdom of God.

So, keep leaning in to your Home Base Habits, and use your Fully Nourished Check-Ins even when life feels chaotic. These practices will anchor you, reminding you that food freedom isn't a destination—it's a way of life that empowers you to serve others and honor God. Remember, this book is your guide, designed to be revisited as you grow. Come back to the sections that resonate or lead you to areas that need deeper work. Each time you do, you'll find fresh insights to support you on your journey.

And finally, don't forget that you're never walking this road alone. In moments of uncertainty, when the path seems unclear or your strength falters, turn to the One who called you here. His grace will carry you through the rough patches, and his love will remind you that you are already enough—just as you are (Zeph. 3:17).

For added encouragement and support, I invite you to visit https://GraceFilledPlate.com/fnbonus/, if you have not already done so, to learn more about our online community so you can surround yourself with others who understand this journey. We lift each other up, share insights, and celebrate victories together. You're warmly welcomed to walk this path with us, knowing that together we're stronger, grounded in faith, and committed to living in true food freedom.

As you continue, my prayer is that you experience the fullness of God's presence in every area of your life. May his presence guide your every step and his love fill every corner of your heart, and may you always remember that true freedom is found in Christ alone.

ACKNOWLEDGMENTS

To my heavenly Father, who loved me before I took my first breath. It was your grace that changed me. May all who find freedom through this book give you the glory.

To my Savior, Jesus Christ, who understands what it is like to struggle and whose blood allows me to come boldly to the throne of grace to receive mercy and help in times of need.

And to the Holy Spirit, whose gentle whisperings have led me to do more than I could ask, imagine, or think.

To my husband, Doug, my best friend and the love of my life: Thank you for your unwavering support and belief in me, and for teaching me what unconditional love truly is.

To my daughter, who inspires me every day. I am so proud of the remarkable person you are becoming.

To my parents, who have supported every crazy dream I've had and picked me up when things didn't go as planned.

To my mother-in-love, Felicia, who has sat with me through some of the hardest times in my life.

To my late Grandma Brown, who hid her hard-earned money behind a picture frame so her grandkids could chase their dreams. That seed investment launched Grace Filled Plate.

In loving memory of Carol Burmood: Thank you for being the literal hands and feet of Jesus in my life.

To Blythe Daniel, my incredible agent: Thank you for believing in me and pushing me to become a better writer.

To the amazing team at Revell, including Kelsey Bowen, Brianna DeWitt, Anne Van Solkema, and Lindsey Spoolstra: Thank you for catching my vision and making it come to life. I am beyond grateful!

To Cheri Gregory, my writing coach: Your encouragement and reminders to be gentle with myself during this process were such a gift.

To Aubrey Golbek, RD: Thank you for reviewing the nutrition-centric chapters with your grace- and joy-filled perspective.

To my manuscript development team: Audrey Pearson, Mara Madarász, Lyndsi Irwin, Lisa Hall, Margaret Davis, Marge Halterman, Julie M., Nancy A., Suzanne Hartley, Patti Long, Rebecca Masney, Kim Volk, Elmaret Fourie, Debbie B., Cathy D., Meghan C., Shari T., Deanna T., Kristine M., Kendra, and all the other women who participated. Thank you for previewing this book and offering your valuable insights.

To my business buddies: Lisa Yvonne, Corina Holden, Kati Kiefer, Ruthie Gray, and Kristine Bolt. Your camaraderie has been a joy and a blessing.

To Ginger Perkins: Your faithful support and steadfast presence in both Grace Filled Plate and Platinum have been a priceless gift. You've poured your heart and soul into this ministry as if it were your own, and your reliability, creativity, and care have touched more lives than you know. I'm deeply grateful for the way you've walked beside me every step of the way.

To the Grace Filled Plate Support Team: Erin, Karen, Suzanne, Sophia, and Lyndsie. Thank you for all you do.

To my Grace Filled Plate Platinum members: You are the ones who have implemented these strategies and proven their effectiveness. Thank you for your trust, your feedback, and for inspiring me every step of the way.

Finally, to anyone whose name I may have unintentionally forgotten, please know that your support and encouragement have been deeply appreciated and have played a meaningful role in this journey. I am truly grateful for you.

This book exists because of all of you. Thank you from the bottom of my heart.

APPENDIX

Welcome to the appendix—a space designed to give you extra support as you live out the grace-filled habits you've learned. You'll find practical tools like habit-adjustment strategies, lists of common limiting beliefs and sabotaging thoughts, and helpful mindset shifts to keep you moving forward when things get tough. You'll also discover food quality guides to help you take small steps toward nourishment, plus a grace-based approach to understanding emotional eating.

Think of this as your follow-through toolbox—here when you need clarity, encouragement, or a fresh dose of motivation. Whether you're adjusting a habit, confronting a limiting belief, or simply navigating a hard day, these resources are here to support you with truth, wisdom, and grace.

HOW TO ADJUST A HABIT

When should you consider adjusting a habit? If your confidence in sticking with a habit is less than an 8 out of 10, or if you find your current habit isn't working as intended, it's time to make a shift. Adjusting your habit in one of the following three ways can make it more doable, sustainable, and ultimately more effective. By setting realistic expectations, you'll achieve the consistency needed to adopt long-term habits and, in turn, build your confidence in the change process.

1. **Reduce the frequency.**
   If your habit feels overwhelming, try reducing how often you aim to complete it. For example:
   - Instead of eating vegetables at both lunch and dinner, try focusing on adding them to just one meal a day.
   - If walking five days a week is too much, aim for three days instead.
   - Waiting for hunger before every meal might feel too rigid, so try practicing this with one meal a day that feels more flexible.

2. **Lessen the intensity.**
   If your habit feels too difficult, consider reducing its intensity. For example:
   - Aim for three servings of vegetables a day rather than five.
   - Shorten your walking routine from thirty minutes to fifteen minutes.
   - If sitting with hunger for thirty minutes feels too hard, try reducing it to fifteen minutes.

3. **Add flexibility.**
   When a habit feels too rigid, introduce more flexibility to make it manageable. For example:
   - Instead of committing to eating vegetables at every meal, aim for most meals.
   - Rather than sticking to a strict Monday, Wednesday, and Friday walking routine, aim to walk three days a week whenever it works for you.
   - If eating only when you're hungry is too strict, try practicing it once a day.

As these examples show, small adjustments can make a big difference, transforming your habits into something more achievable. Keep experimenting until you find a variation that feels right for you!

LIST OF LIMITING BELIEFS

General

I'm not good enough.

I don't have what it takes.

I'm too old/young.

I don't deserve success/happiness.

I cannot trust others.

I'm not smart enough.

I'm not worthy of love.

I can't change my circumstances.

I'll never be successful.

I don't belong anywhere.

I'm not interesting to others.

I'm bound to fail.

I must not make mistakes.

People will always let me down.

I can't handle pressure or stress.

I shouldn't be too ambitious.

I can't do things on my own.

I'm destined to be unhappy.

I must please everyone to be liked.

I'm not the type of person who succeeds.

I can't be honest about my feelings.

I must keep my problems to myself.

I don't have the skills to adapt or learn new things.

Food Freedom Specific

I can't lose weight no matter what I try.

Healthy food isn't tasty.

I don't like to cook.

I don't have the willpower to stick to a diet.

I'm too busy to cook or prepare healthy meals.

It's too expensive to eat healthily.

I have bad genetics, so dieting won't help.

I can't control myself around food.

I don't have time to exercise.

Losing weight is too hard.

I don't like vegetables.

I deserve to eat whatever I want.

I'm too old to change my eating habits.

I need to eat a lot to feel satisfied.

I'll always be overweight.

I can't eat leftovers.

Dieting means feeling hungry all the time.

I can't maintain weight loss long-term.

I need food to cope with stress or emotions.

I can't make better choices because my family won't.

LIST OF SABOTAGING THOUGHTS

I'll make up for it later.

I'll do better tomorrow.

I'll be better once the holidays are over.

It's healthy, so it's okay.

I think I'm hungry.

I'm not that full.

It's just this once.

I've been doing so well; it's okay.

I deserve to have this.

Everyone else is having it.

I have to eat this now; I might not get the chance again.

I can't waste food.

I'll stop eating sugar tomorrow.

It's been a hard day.

It's not fair that I can't have it.

I'll never lose weight anyway.

I lost weight, so I have more wiggle room.

It's a special day.

It's free.

I don't care.

I don't want to disappoint.

I'll start on Monday.

Just one won't hurt.

I can burn this off at the gym.

Life is too short not to indulge.

I need a treat to cheer myself up.

I've already messed up today, so I might as well continue.

I worked hard today, so I earned this.

I've always been this way.

This is just how I am.

It's too hard.

Why bother; I just keep failing.

It costs too much to eat healthily.

If I don't eat a lot now, I'll be hungry later.

Calories don't count today.

I've failed every time; I may as well quit now.

I deserve a reward for all the good choices I've made.

I'm too tired to make something healthy.

THE CONTINUUM OF FOOD QUALITY

As you've learned, sustainable change happens progressively. When it comes to transitioning to more whole foods and healthier choices, making a drastic leap from A to Z can feel overwhelming and be counterproductive. Instead, small, manageable adaptations allow you to build lasting habits that remain doable, even on tough days.

Below is a continuum of simple food swaps that make eating healthier more accessible. Use these as inspiration, or find where you currently are on the chart and use the options to help you brainstorm one step forward toward more nutritious eating.

Food Quality Hack: Take One Step to the Right

bottled smoothie	store-bought fresh smoothie	homemade smoothie with fruit	homemade smoothie with fruit and spinach
packaged sweetened oatmeal	packaged unsweetened oatmeal	homemade oats with honey or fruit	steel-cut oats with fresh fruit
sugary breakfast cereal	whole grain cereal	homemade granola	plain oatmeal with nuts and fruit
white bread	store-bought whole wheat bread	homemade whole grain bread	sprouted grain bread
prepackaged deli meats	low-sodium deli meats	grilled chicken or turkey slices	grilled chicken or turkey breast
packaged mac and cheese	packaged whole grain mac and cheese	homemade mac and cheese with whole wheat pasta	baked spaghetti squash with cheese sauce
fast-food fried chicken	homemade fried chicken	homemade breaded and baked chicken	grilled chicken
fast-food hamburger	fast-food grilled chicken sandwich	homemade hamburger	homemade hamburger with lean meat and whole grain bun
fast-food french fries	frozen french fries cooked at home	frozen french fries baked at home	homemade oven fries made from whole potatoes
fast-food pizza	store-bought pizza	homemade pizza with whole grain crust	cauliflower crust pizza with veggies

sugary store-bought salad dressing	low-sugar store-bought salad dressing	homemade vinaigrette	olive oil with lemon or vinegar
canned soup	reduced-sodium canned soup	homemade soup	homemade vegetable soup with lean protein
potato chips	baked potato chips	air-popped popcorn	kale or sweet potato chips
canned fruit in syrup	canned fruit in juice	fresh fruit with yogurt	fresh, whole fruit
packaged snack bars	homemade energy bites	homemade snack bars with nuts and seeds	nuts, seeds, and fresh fruit
store-bought cookies	homemade cookies with less sugar	Homemade cookies with whole grain flour	fruit with nuts or seeds
ice cream	frozen yogurt	fruit-based frozen dessert	fresh fruit with Greek yogurt
soda	low-sugar drink	sparkling water with fruit	water or herbal tea

WHAT TO DO WHEN YOU'RE EMOTIONAL EATING

It's something we all experience: We're eating, but we're not hungry. There's no hunger, yet the hand-to-mouth cycle continues: chew, chew, chew . . . rinse and repeat. Maybe it's a box of cereal or a bag of chips, and, deep down, you know that food isn't what you really need, but it's what feels familiar at the moment. The stress, exhaustion, boredom, disappointment, or frustration you're feeling seems unbearable, and zoning out with food, even if only for a moment, feels like the easiest solution.

Emotional eating has layers. On the surface, it may seem like a simple urge, but there are deeper reasons driving the behavior. The key to overcoming emotional eating is understanding both the practical and emotional causes that lead you to reach for food. In this section, we'll take a top-down approach, starting with the simplest adjustments and working toward uncovering deeper emotional triggers.

What Is Emotional Eating?

Emotional eating occurs when you eat to soothe or feed your emotions rather than to fuel your body.

It's important to remember that this can look different in various situations. For example, enjoying cake at a birthday party or having popcorn during a movie night are forms of emotional eating, but they're often done in the spirit of celebration and connection. Occasional emotional eating isn't something to stress over— acknowledge it and move forward. It's when emotional eating becomes habitual or tied to negative emotions like stress or anger that we need to dig deeper for solutions.

When Emotional Eating Becomes a Problem

If food is your go-to for stress relief, boredom, or managing emotions, it's time to explore what's really going on. Constantly using food as a coping mechanism can prevent you from living fully. It becomes a barrier to addressing your emotional or spiritual needs that are crying out for attention.

Here, we'll break down a two-step process to help you overcome emotional eating. While this isn't an overnight fix, these steps will guide you toward identifying your core emotional triggers and help you develop healthier responses.

Step 1: Identify the Why

When you feel the urge to emotionally eat, pause for a moment before reaching for food. Set a timer for one to three minutes and ask yourself the following questions:

- Why am I choosing this food right now?
- What do I hope to gain from this experience?
- What am I avoiding, and what am I afraid will happen if I don't eat?

It's normal to feel that eating is the quickest way to ease discomfort, but recognizing the underlying emotion can help you take compassionate steps toward a healthier approach.

There are three parts of emotional eating: physical, emotional, and spiritual needs. Sometimes a simple solution like rest or a short walk can make all the difference. Other times you might need to address deeper emotional wounds or unmet spiritual needs. Be honest with yourself and allow grace as you uncover these layers.

Step 2: Meet the True Need

Once you've identified why you're turning to food, it's time to shift your response. Food might have been your "knight in shining armor" for a long time, but you've grown beyond needing food to be your emotional rescuer. You are now capable of meeting your true needs in healthier, more sustainable ways.

Meeting your true needs might look like this:

- If you're exhausted, rest. Find small moments throughout the day to rest your mind and body, perhaps by going to bed earlier, taking a short walk, or finding fifteen minutes of quiet time.
- If you're bored, get creative. Engage in activities that bring you joy or mental stimulation, like reading, crafting, or organizing. It's about finding something that fills you up rather than drains you.
- If you're stressed, address it. Stress eating often provides temporary relief but adds to your long-term stress. Identify the sources of your stress and seek healthier outlets like journaling, prayer, or talking to a friend.

At times, emotional eating can stem from a deep need for *comfort*. It's tempting to turn to food when life feels overwhelming, but true comfort comes from resting in God's peace. Learning how to use your desire to eat as a trigger to turn to the Lord will allow you to make friends with the desire and use it for your good and his glory!

BRANDICE LARDNER

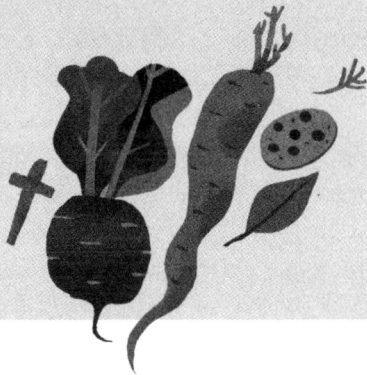

is a personal trainer, nutrition coach, and owner and author of Grace Filled Plate, which she founded in 2017. She has helped hundreds of women through one-on-one and group coaching programs, teaching them how to find food freedom by meeting their physical, emotional, and spiritual needs. She's appeared on numerous podcasts, including *Do It Scared with Ruth Soukup*, and has been featured as a guest expert on MyFitnessPal, MapMyRun, TLC Online, and Women's Running. She lives in Clearwater, Florida, with her family.

Connect with Brandice:

🌐 GraceFilledPlate.com

f @GraceFilledPlate

📷 @BrandiceLardner

A Note from the Publisher

Dear Reader,

Thank you for selecting a Revell book! We're so happy to be part of your life through this work.

Revell's mission is to publish books that offer hope and help for meeting life's challenges, and that bring comfort and inspiration. We know that the right words at the right time can make all the difference; it is our goal with every title to provide just the words you need.

We believe in building lasting relationships with readers, and we'd love to get to know you better. If you have any feedback, questions, or just want to chat about your experience reading this book, please email us directly at publisher@revellbooks.com. Your insights are incredibly important to us, and it would be our pleasure to hear how we can better serve you.

We look forward to hearing from you and having the chance to enhance your experience with Revell Books.

The Publishing Team at Revell Books
A Division of Baker Publishing Group
publisher@revellbooks.com

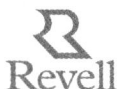

Revell